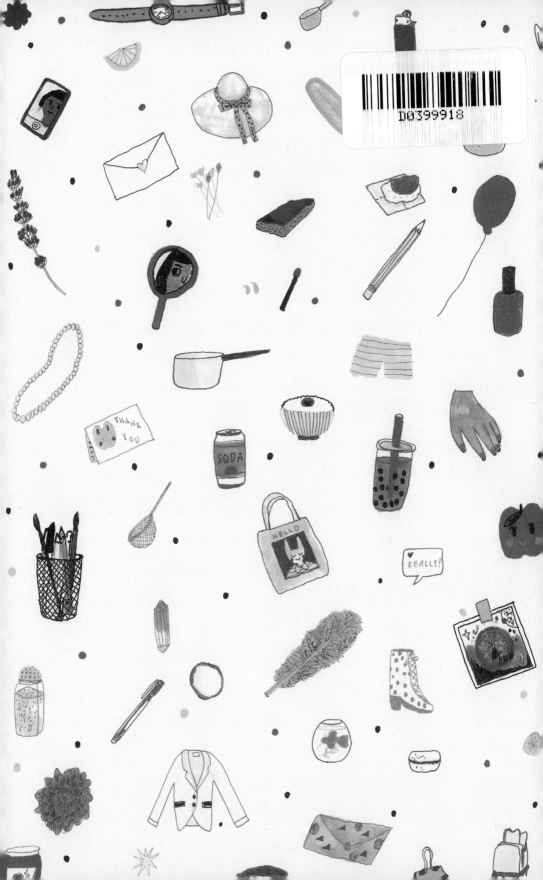

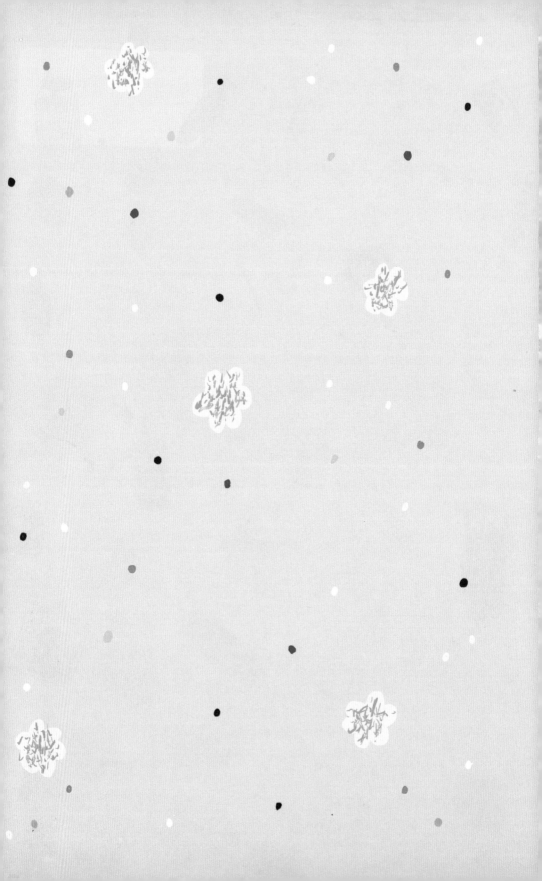

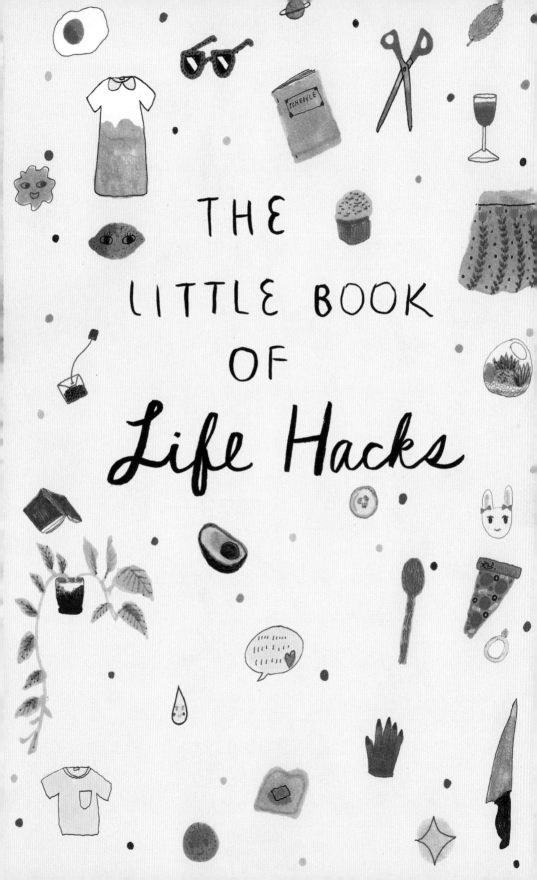

THE
LITTLE BOOK
OF
Life Hacks

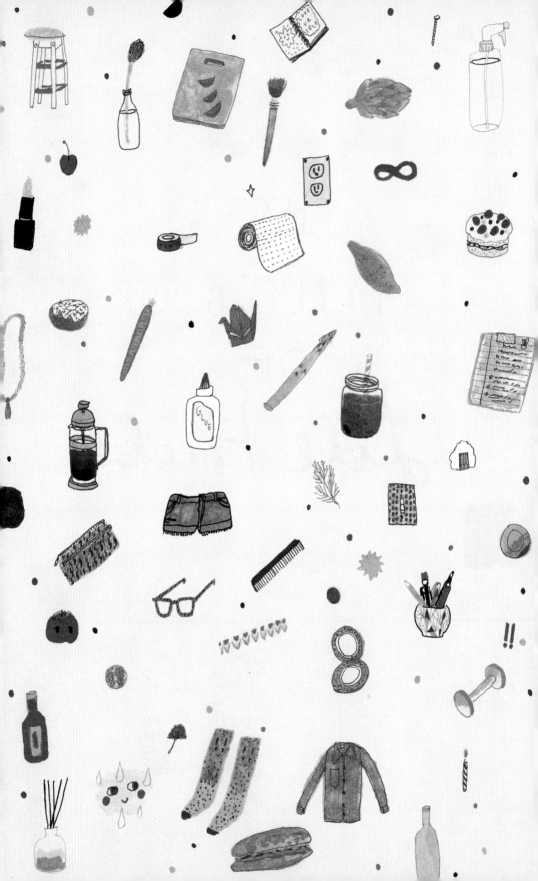

THE
LITTLE
BOOK OF
Life Hacks

How to make Your Life
HAPPIER, HEALTHIER,
and MORE BEAUTIFUL

YUMI SAKUGAWA

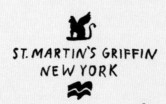

ST. MARTIN'S GRIFFIN
NEW YORK

THE LITTLE BOOK OF LIFE HACKS. COPYRIGHT © 2017 BY YUMI SAKUGAWA.
ALL RIGHTS RESERVED. PRINTED IN USA. FOR INFORMATION, ADDRESS
ST. MARTIN'S PRESS, 175 FIFTH AVENUE, NEW YORK, N.Y. 10010.

www.stmartins.com

PORTIONS OF THIS BOOK PREVIOUSLY APPEARED ON WonderHowTo.com
IN A SLIGHTLY DIFFERENT FORM.

THE LIBRARY OF CONGRESS CATALOGING-IN-PUBLICATION DATA IS
AVAILABLE UPON REQUEST.

ISBN 978-1-250-09225-0 (PAPER OVER BOARD)
ISBN 978-1-250-09226-7 (E-BOOK)

OUR BOOKS MAY BE PURCHASED IN BULK FOR PROMOTIONAL,
EDUCATIONAL, OR BUSINESS USE. PLEASE CONTACT YOUR LOCAL
BOOKSELLER OR THE MACMILLAN CORPORATE AND PREMIUM
SALES DEPARTMENT AT 1-800-221-7945, EXTENSION 5442, OR BY
E-MAIL AT MACMILLANSPECIALMARKETS@MACMILLAN.COM.

FIRST EDITION: MAY 2017

10 9 8 7 6 5 4

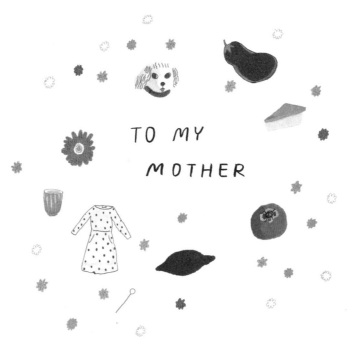

TO MY
MOTHER

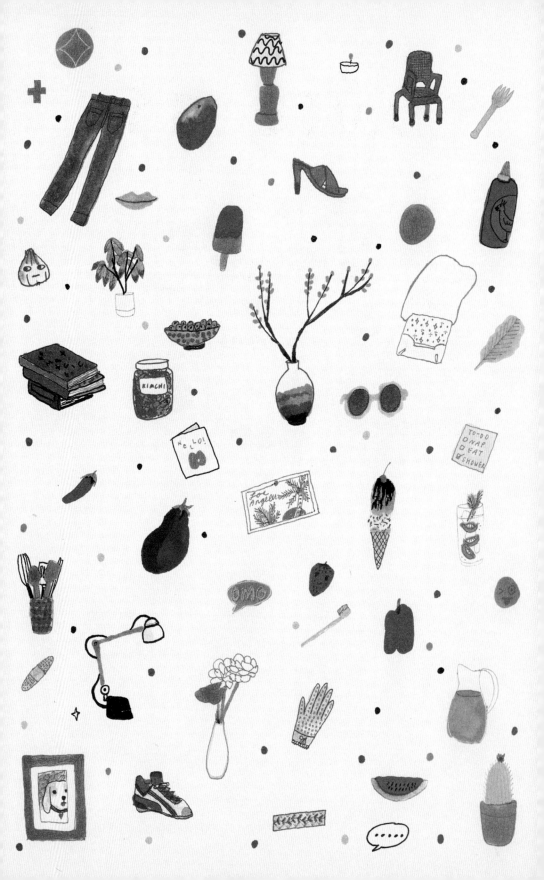

CONTENTS

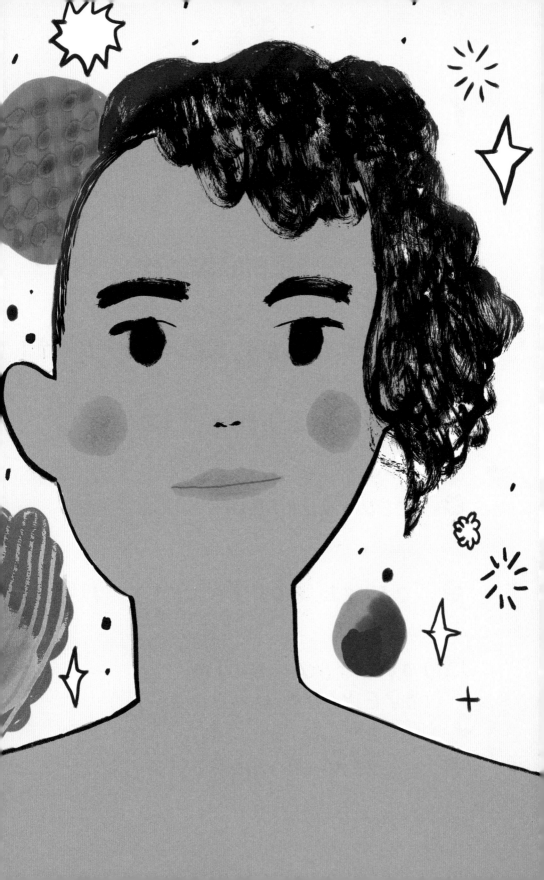

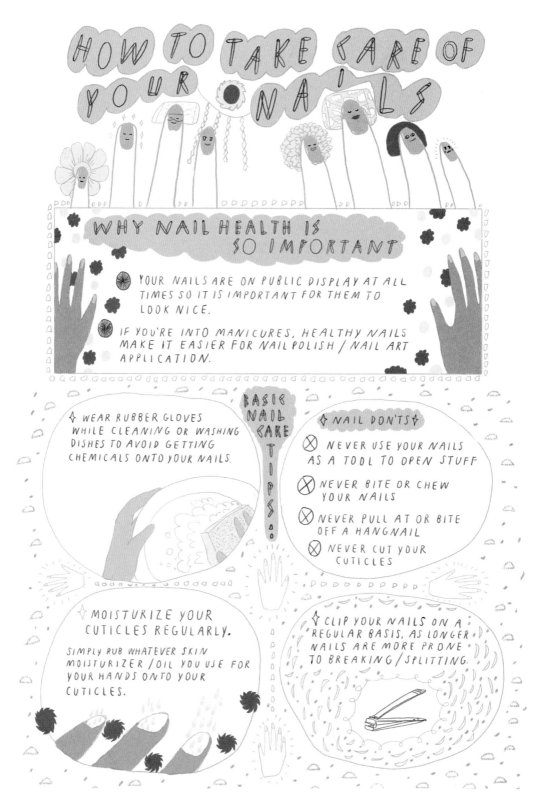

HOW TO TAKE CARE OF YOUR NAILS

WHY NAIL HEALTH IS SO IMPORTANT

- YOUR NAILS ARE ON PUBLIC DISPLAY AT ALL TIMES SO IT IS IMPORTANT FOR THEM TO LOOK NICE.

- IF YOU'RE INTO MANICURES, HEALTHY NAILS MAKE IT EASIER FOR NAIL POLISH / NAIL ART APPLICATION.

BASIC NAIL CARE TIPS

✦ WEAR RUBBER GLOVES WHILE CLEANING OR WASHING DISHES TO AVOID GETTING CHEMICALS ONTO YOUR NAILS.

✦ NAIL DON'TS ✦

- ⊗ NEVER USE YOUR NAILS AS A TOOL TO OPEN STUFF
- ⊗ NEVER BITE OR CHEW YOUR NAILS
- ⊗ NEVER PULL AT OR BITE OFF A HANGNAIL
- ⊗ NEVER CUT YOUR CUTICLES

✦ MOISTURIZE YOUR CUTICLES REGULARLY.

SIMPLY RUB WHATEVER SKIN MOISTURIZER / OIL YOU USE FOR YOUR HANDS ONTO YOUR CUTICLES.

✦ CLIP YOUR NAILS ON A REGULAR BASIS, AS LONGER NAILS ARE MORE PRONE TO BREAKING / SPLITTING.

DiY BEAUTIFUL

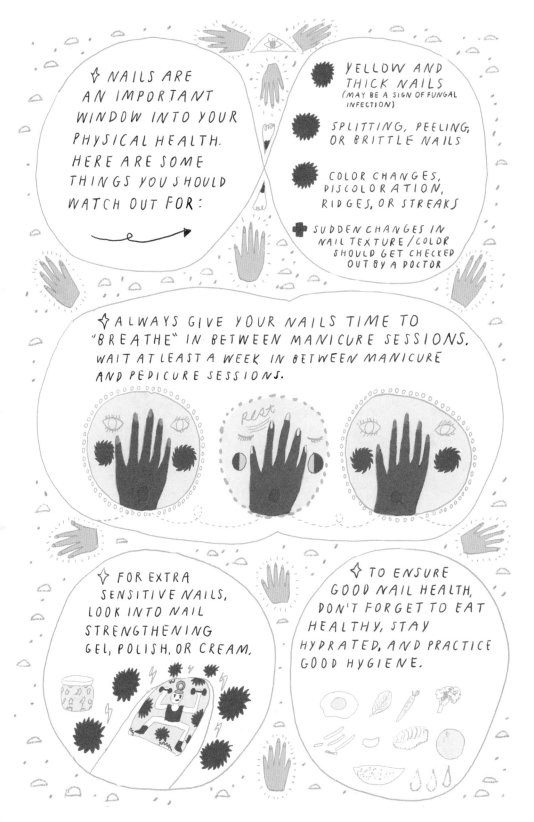

✡ NAILS ARE AN IMPORTANT WINDOW INTO YOUR PHYSICAL HEALTH. HERE ARE SOME THINGS YOU SHOULD WATCH OUT FOR:

YELLOW AND THICK NAILS (MAY BE A SIGN OF FUNGAL INFECTION)

SPLITTING, PEELING, OR BRITTLE NAILS

COLOR CHANGES, DISCOLORATION, RIDGES, OR STREAKS

✚ SUDDEN CHANGES IN NAIL TEXTURE/COLOR SHOULD GET CHECKED OUT BY A DOCTOR

✡ ALWAYS GIVE YOUR NAILS TIME TO "BREATHE" IN BETWEEN MANICURE SESSIONS. WAIT AT LEAST A WEEK IN BETWEEN MANICURE AND PEDICURE SESSIONS.

Rest

✡ FOR EXTRA SENSITIVE NAILS, LOOK INTO NAIL STRENGTHENING GEL, POLISH, OR CREAM.

✡ TO ENSURE GOOD NAIL HEALTH, DON'T FORGET TO EAT HEALTHY, STAY HYDRATED, AND PRACTICE GOOD HYGIENE.

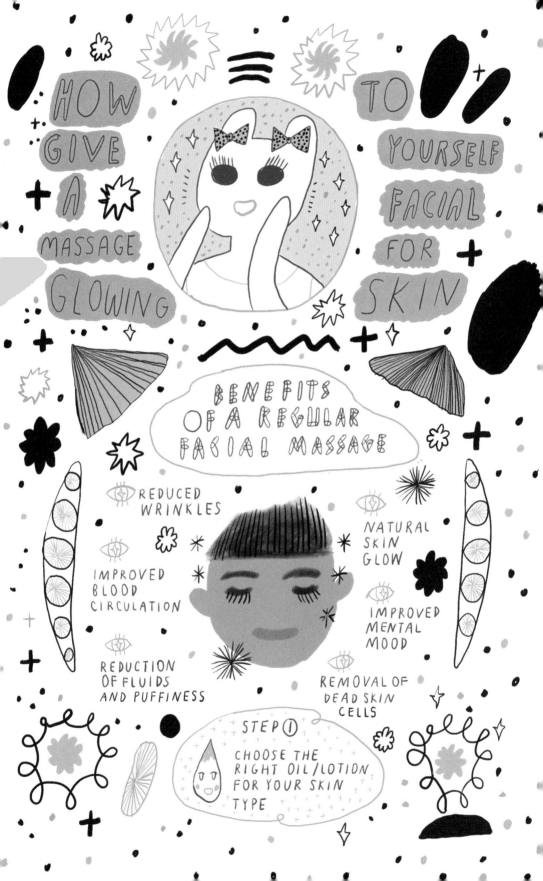

HOW TO GIVE YOURSELF A FACIAL MASSAGE FOR GLOWING SKIN

BENEFITS OF A REGULAR FACIAL MASSAGE

- REDUCED WRINKLES
- IMPROVED BLOOD CIRCULATION
- REDUCTION OF FLUIDS AND PUFFINESS
- NATURAL SKIN GLOW
- IMPROVED MENTAL MOOD
- REMOVAL OF DEAD SKIN CELLS

STEP ①
CHOOSE THE RIGHT OIL/LOTION FOR YOUR SKIN TYPE

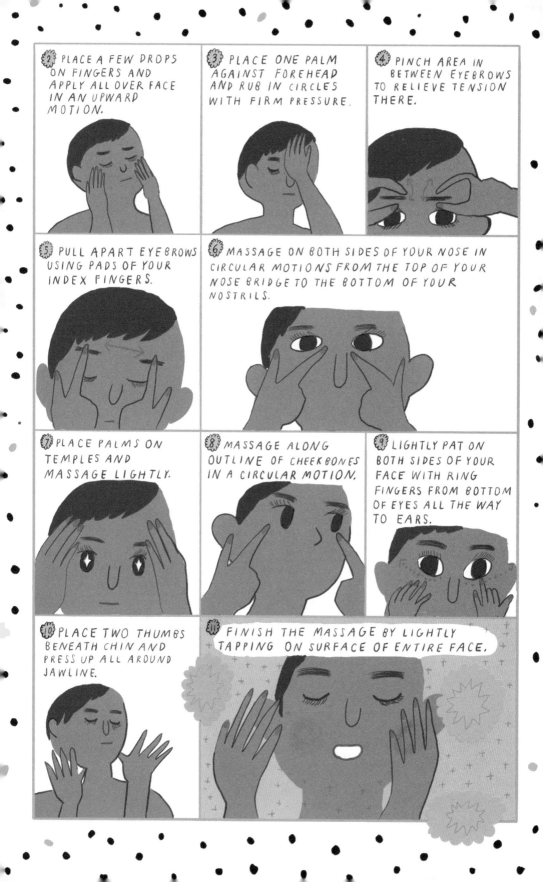

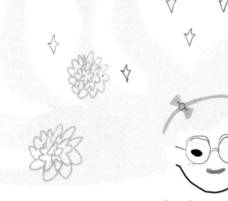

TIPS FOR HAVING HEALTHY & ATTRACTIVE HAIR

SPECIAL TREATMENTS YOU CAN GIVE YOUR HAIR ONCE A WEEK

TREATMENT 1

✧ GREAT FOR ADDING MORE SHINE, LUSTER, AND BODY TO DRY OR DULL HAIR ✧

MASH A RIPE AVOCADO (PEELED AND PITTED) AND APPLY TO WET HAIR. LEAVE ON FOR 20 MINUTES AND RINSE OUT.

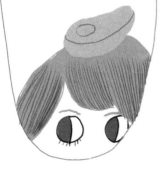

TREATMENT 2

✧ GREAT FOR BALANCING HAIR AND SCALP pH ✧

MAKE A TONIC OUT OF 1 PART APPLE CIDER VINEGAR AND 2 PARTS VERY WARM WATER. POUR OVER HEAD AND MASSAGE INTO SCALP. LET SIT FOR 15 MINUTES AND WASH HAIR AFTERWARD.

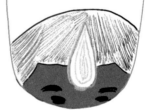

TREATMENT 3

✧ GREAT FOR TREATING DRY, BRITTLE HAIR ✧

DAMPEN HAIR WITH WARM WATER, APPLY MAYONNAISE TO HAIR AS YOU WOULD WITH HAIR CONDITIONER. WRAP HAIR WITH PLASTIC WRAP OR A PLASTIC SHOWER CAP. LEAVE ON FOR 20 MINUTES. WASH OUT IN SHOWER WITH DILUTED SHAMPOO.

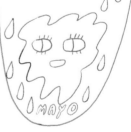

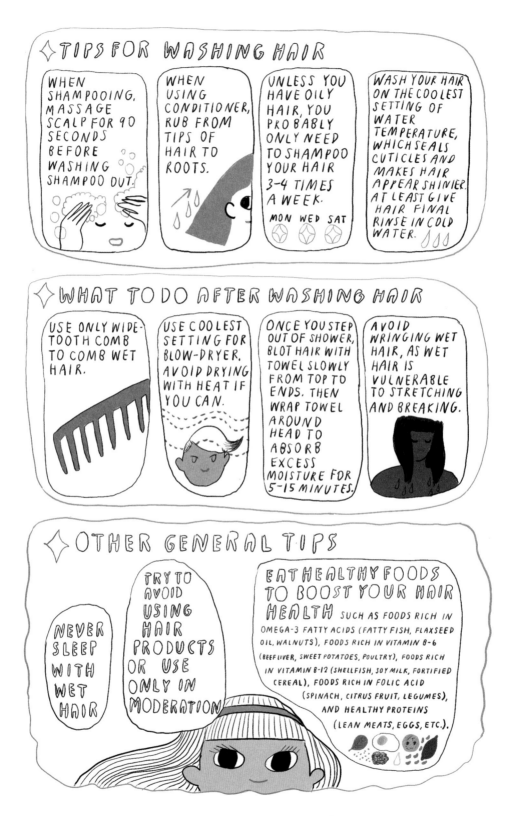

◇ TIPS FOR WASHING HAIR

WHEN SHAMPOOING, MASSAGE SCALP FOR 90 SECONDS BEFORE WASHING SHAMPOO OUT.

WHEN USING CONDITIONER, RUB FROM TIPS OF HAIR TO ROOTS.

UNLESS YOU HAVE OILY HAIR, YOU PROBABLY ONLY NEED TO SHAMPOO YOUR HAIR 3-4 TIMES A WEEK.
MON WED SAT

WASH YOUR HAIR ON THE COOLEST SETTING OF WATER TEMPERATURE, WHICH SEALS CUTICLES AND MAKES HAIR APPEAR SHINIER. AT LEAST GIVE HAIR FINAL RINSE IN COLD WATER.

◇ WHAT TO DO AFTER WASHING HAIR

USE ONLY WIDE-TOOTH COMB TO COMB WET HAIR.

USE COOLEST SETTING FOR BLOW-DRYER. AVOID DRYING WITH HEAT IF YOU CAN.

ONCE YOU STEP OUT OF SHOWER, BLOT HAIR WITH TOWEL SLOWLY FROM TOP TO ENDS. THEN WRAP TOWEL AROUND HEAD TO ABSORB EXCESS MOISTURE FOR 5-15 MINUTES.

AVOID WRINGING WET HAIR, AS WET HAIR IS VULNERABLE TO STRETCHING AND BREAKING.

◇ OTHER GENERAL TIPS

NEVER SLEEP WITH WET HAIR

TRY TO AVOID USING HAIR PRODUCTS OR USE ONLY IN MODERATION

EAT HEALTHY FOODS TO BOOST YOUR HAIR HEALTH SUCH AS FOODS RICH IN OMEGA-3 FATTY ACIDS (FATTY FISH, FLAXSEED OIL, WALNUTS), FOODS RICH IN VITAMIN B-6 (BEEF LIVER, SWEET POTATOES, POULTRY), FOODS RICH IN VITAMIN B-12 (SHELLFISH, SOY MILK, FORTIFIED CEREAL), FOODS RICH IN FOLIC ACID (SPINACH, CITRUS FRUIT, LEGUMES), AND HEALTHY PROTEINS (LEAN MEATS, EGGS, ETC.).

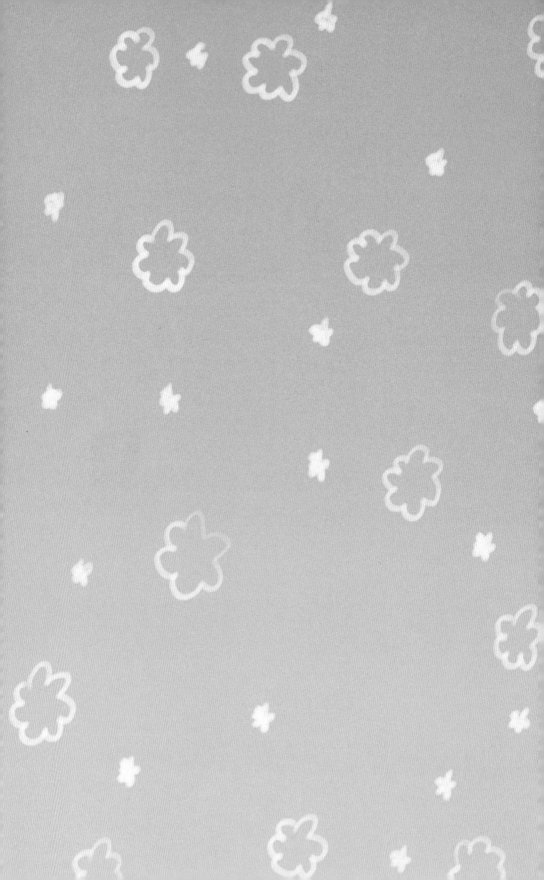

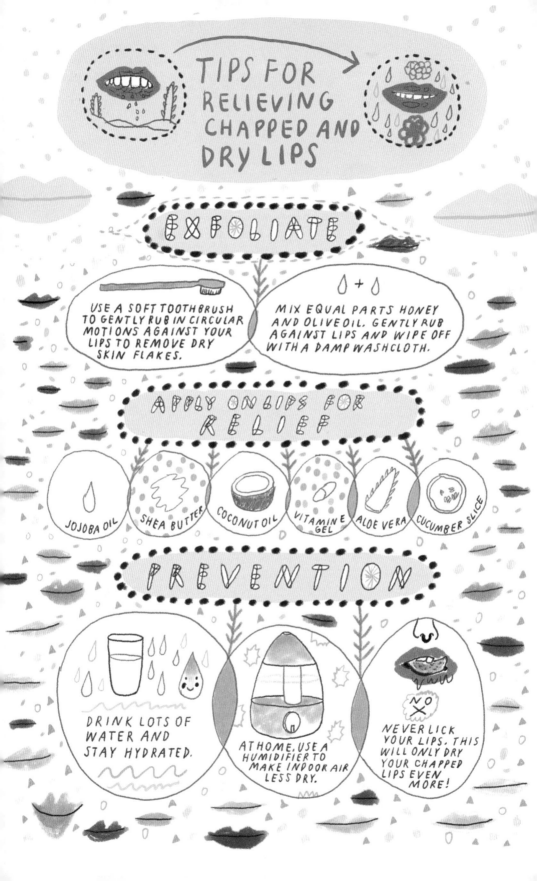

HOW TO MAKE LIPSTICK OUT OF CRAYONS

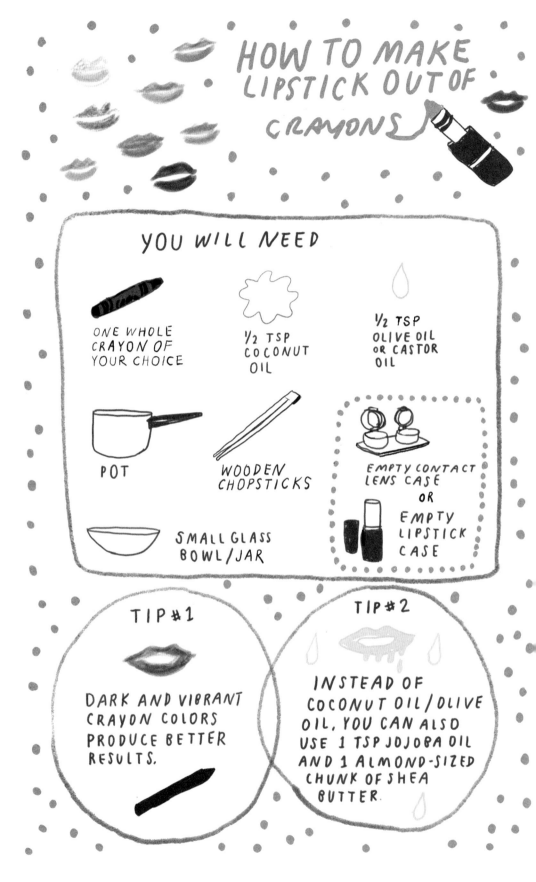

YOU WILL NEED

ONE WHOLE CRAYON OF YOUR CHOICE

½ TSP COCONUT OIL

½ TSP OLIVE OIL OR CASTOR OIL

POT

WOODEN CHOPSTICKS

EMPTY CONTACT LENS CASE

OR

EMPTY LIPSTICK CASE

SMALL GLASS BOWL/JAR

TIP #1

DARK AND VIBRANT CRAYON COLORS PRODUCE BETTER RESULTS.

TIP #2

INSTEAD OF COCONUT OIL/OLIVE OIL, YOU CAN ALSO USE 1 TSP JOJOBA OIL AND 1 ALMOND-SIZED CHUNK OF SHEA BUTTER.

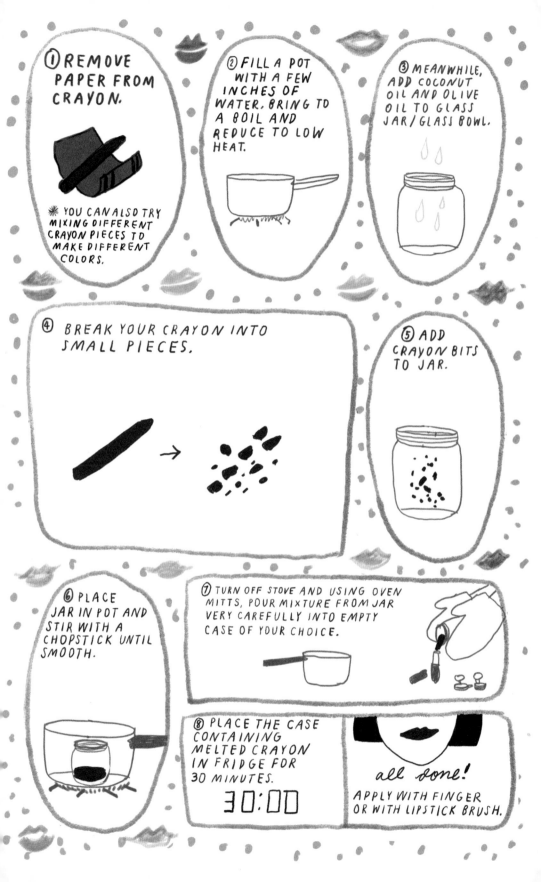

① REMOVE PAPER FROM CRAYON.

✳ YOU CAN ALSO TRY MIXING DIFFERENT CRAYON PIECES TO MAKE DIFFERENT COLORS.

② FILL A POT WITH A FEW INCHES OF WATER, BRING TO A BOIL AND REDUCE TO LOW HEAT.

③ MEANWHILE, ADD COCONUT OIL AND OLIVE OIL TO GLASS JAR/GLASS BOWL.

④ BREAK YOUR CRAYON INTO SMALL PIECES.

⑤ ADD CRAYON BITS TO JAR.

⑥ PLACE JAR IN POT AND STIR WITH A CHOPSTICK UNTIL SMOOTH.

⑦ TURN OFF STOVE AND USING OVEN MITTS, POUR MIXTURE FROM JAR VERY CAREFULLY INTO EMPTY CASE OF YOUR CHOICE.

⑧ PLACE THE CASE CONTAINING MELTED CRAYON IN FRIDGE FOR 30 MINUTES.

30:00

all done!

APPLY WITH FINGER OR WITH LIPSTICK BRUSH.

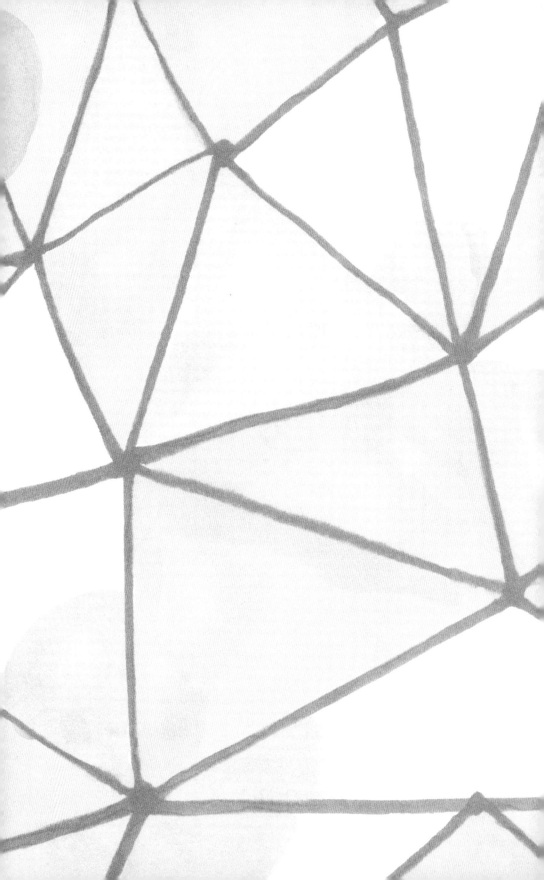

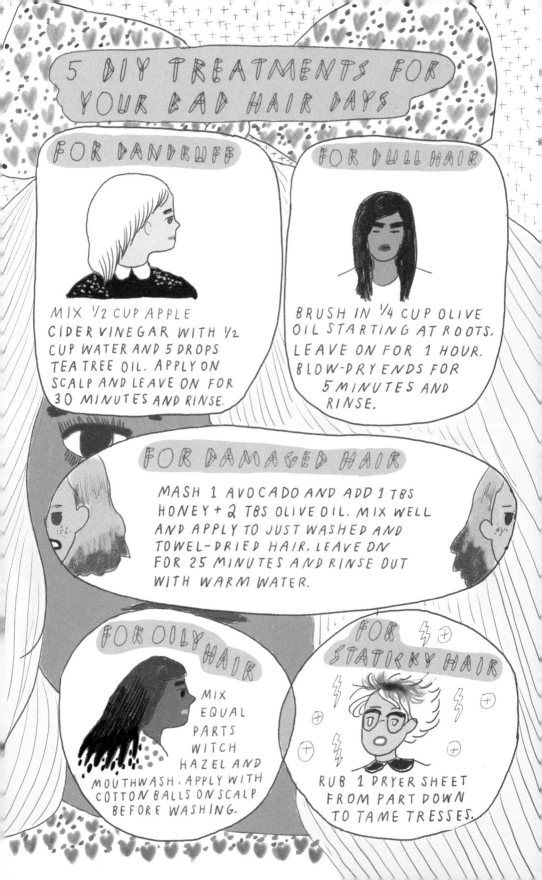

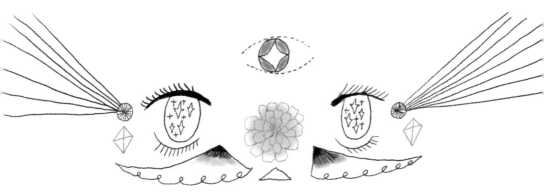

8 HOME REMEDIES FOR RELIEVING DARK CIRCLES UNDER YOUR EYES

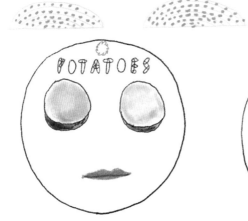

POTATOES

○ PLACE COLD POTATO SLICES ON TOP OF YOUR CLOSED EYES FOR 10-15 MINUTES.

COLD METAL SPOONS

○ LAY ROUNDED SIDES AGAINST EYES FOR 5-10 MINUTES.

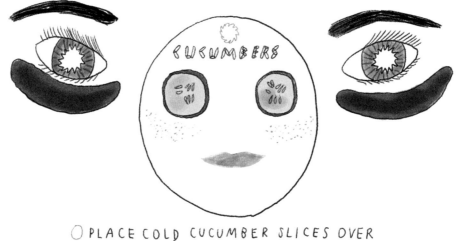

CUCUMBERS

○ PLACE COLD CUCUMBER SLICES OVER EYES FOR 5-10 MINUTES.

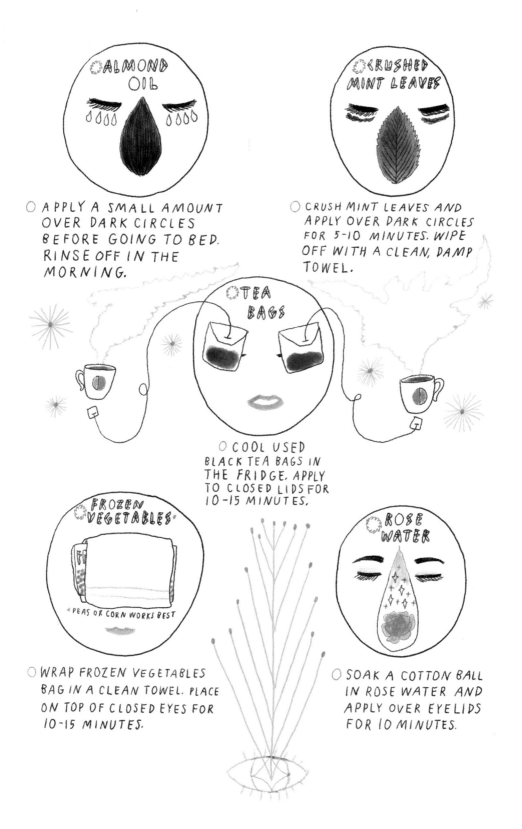

○ ALMOND OIL

○ APPLY A SMALL AMOUNT OVER DARK CIRCLES BEFORE GOING TO BED. RINSE OFF IN THE MORNING.

○ CRUSHED MINT LEAVES

○ CRUSH MINT LEAVES AND APPLY OVER DARK CIRCLES FOR 5-10 MINUTES. WIPE OFF WITH A CLEAN, DAMP TOWEL.

○ TEA BAGS

○ COOL USED BLACK TEA BAGS IN THE FRIDGE. APPLY TO CLOSED LIDS FOR 10-15 MINUTES.

○ FROZEN VEGETABLES

← PEAS OR CORN WORKS BEST

○ WRAP FROZEN VEGETABLES BAG IN A CLEAN TOWEL. PLACE ON TOP OF CLOSED EYES FOR 10-15 MINUTES.

○ ROSE WATER

○ SOAK A COTTON BALL IN ROSE WATER AND APPLY OVER EYELIDS FOR 10 MINUTES.

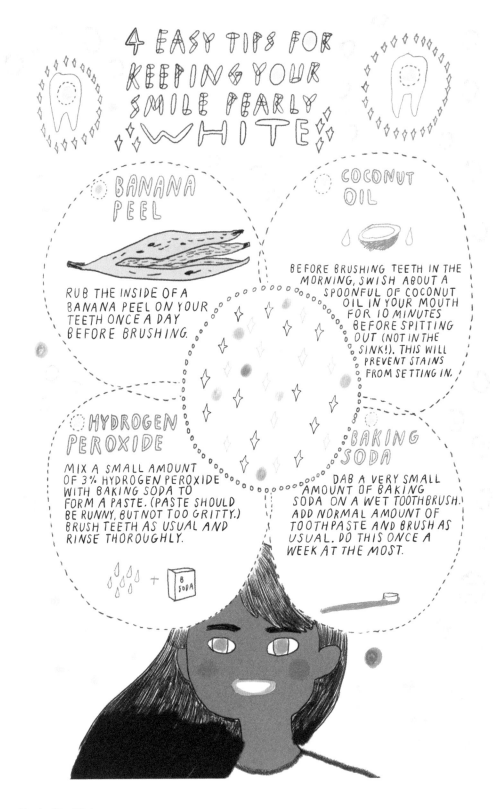

4 EASY TIPS FOR KEEPING YOUR SMILE PEARLY WHITE

BANANA PEEL

RUB THE INSIDE OF A BANANA PEEL ON YOUR TEETH ONCE A DAY BEFORE BRUSHING.

COCONUT OIL

BEFORE BRUSHING TEETH IN THE MORNING, SWISH ABOUT A SPOONFUL OF COCONUT OIL IN YOUR MOUTH FOR 10 MINUTES BEFORE SPITTING OUT (NOT IN THE SINK!). THIS WILL PREVENT STAINS FROM SETTING IN.

HYDROGEN PEROXIDE

MIX A SMALL AMOUNT OF 3% HYDROGEN PEROXIDE WITH BAKING SODA TO FORM A PASTE. (PASTE SHOULD BE RUNNY, BUT NOT TOO GRITTY.) BRUSH TEETH AS USUAL AND RINSE THOROUGHLY.

BAKING SODA

DAB A VERY SMALL AMOUNT OF BAKING SODA ON A WET TOOTHBRUSH. ADD NORMAL AMOUNT OF TOOTHPASTE AND BRUSH AS USUAL. DO THIS ONCE A WEEK AT THE MOST.

OTHER THINGS
YOU CAN DO TO
KEEP YOUR TEETH
PEARLY WHITE

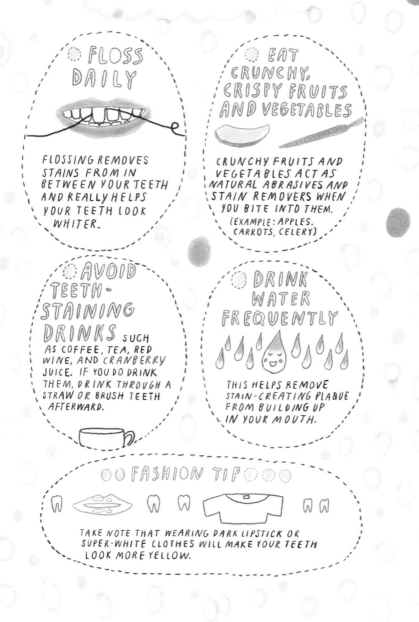

FLOSS DAILY

FLOSSING REMOVES STAINS FROM IN BETWEEN YOUR TEETH AND REALLY HELPS YOUR TEETH LOOK WHITER.

EAT CRUNCHY, CRISPY FRUITS AND VEGETABLES

CRUNCHY FRUITS AND VEGETABLES ACT AS NATURAL ABRASIVES AND STAIN REMOVERS WHEN YOU BITE INTO THEM. (EXAMPLE: APPLES, CARROTS, CELERY)

AVOID TEETH-STAINING DRINKS

SUCH AS COFFEE, TEA, RED WINE, AND CRANBERRY JUICE. IF YOU DO DRINK THEM, DRINK THROUGH A STRAW OR BRUSH TEETH AFTERWARD.

DRINK WATER FREQUENTLY

THIS HELPS REMOVE STAIN-CREATING PLAQUE FROM BUILDING UP IN YOUR MOUTH.

FASHION TIP

TAKE NOTE THAT WEARING DARK LIPSTICK OR SUPER-WHITE CLOTHES WILL MAKE YOUR TEETH LOOK MORE YELLOW.

HOW TO REMOVE EYE MAKEUP THE DIY WAY

PLACE ANY OF THE INGREDIENTS BELOW ON A COTTON SWAB OR Q-TIP AND GENTLY RUB UNTIL EYE MAKEUP IS REMOVED.

YOU CAN ALSO MAKE YOUR OWN EYE MAKEUP REMOVER SOLUTION (SEE BELOW). APPLY WITH A COTTON SWAB.

ALOE VERA GEL

COCONUT OIL

ALMOND OIL

MILK

OLIVE OIL   JOJOBA OIL   GRAPE-SEED OIL

SHEA BUTTER

* YOU CAN ALSO WIPE OFF MAKEUP WITH A CUCUMBER SLICE

RECIPE 1

◊ + ◊

MIX TOGETHER 2 OZ WITCH HAZEL AND 2 OZ OLIVE OIL. STORE IN A GLASS JAR.

RECIPE 2

◊ + ◊ + ◊

MIX TOGETHER 1 CUP DISTILLED WATER, 1/4 TSP CASTILE SOAP, AND 1 TSP OLIVE OIL.

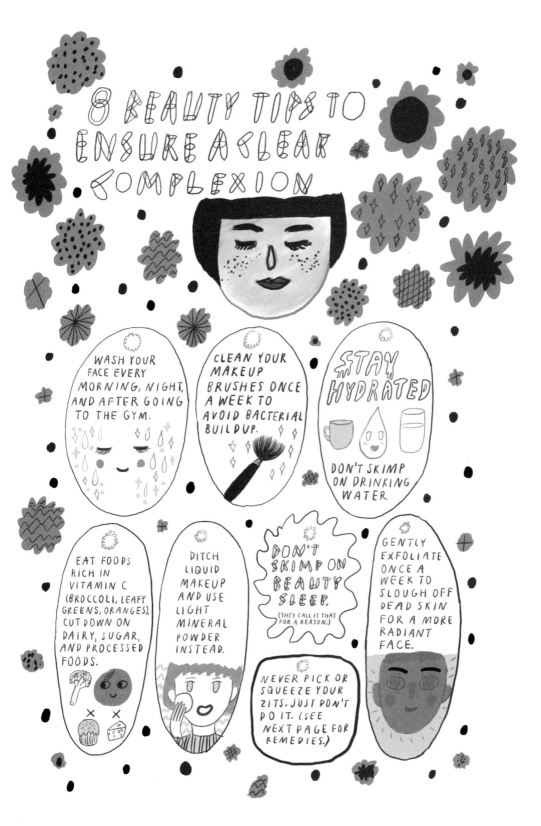

8 BEAUTY TIPS TO ENSURE A CLEAR COMPLEXION

WASH YOUR FACE EVERY MORNING, NIGHT, AND AFTER GOING TO THE GYM.

CLEAN YOUR MAKEUP BRUSHES ONCE A WEEK TO AVOID BACTERIAL BUILDUP.

STAY HYDRATED

DON'T SKIMP ON DRINKING WATER.

EAT FOODS RICH IN VITAMIN C (BROCCOLI, LEAFY GREENS, ORANGES). CUT DOWN ON DAIRY, SUGAR, AND PROCESSED FOODS.

DITCH LIQUID MAKEUP AND USE LIGHT MINERAL POWDER INSTEAD.

DON'T SKIMP ON BEAUTY SLEEP. (THEY CALL IT THAT FOR A REASON.)

NEVER PICK OR SQUEEZE YOUR ZITS. JUST DON'T DO IT. (SEE NEXT PAGE FOR REMEDIES.)

GENTLY EXFOLIATE ONCE A WEEK TO SLOUGH OFF DEAD SKIN FOR A MORE RADIANT FACE.

BONUS: DIY REMEDIES FOR TREATING ZITS

EGG WHITES
SEPARATE EGG WHITE FROM YOLK. APPLY ON FACE FOR 20 MINUTES AND RINSE OFF.

TEA TREE OIL
DAB SMALL AMOUNT ON AFFECTED AREA WITH Q-TIP AND LEAVE ON OVERNIGHT.

HONEY
USE AS FACIAL MASK. REALLY STICKY BUT EFFECTIVE. RAW, UNFILTERED HONEY CONTAINS MORE HEALING PROPERTIES, AND YOU REALLY ONLY NEED ABOUT 1 TSP.

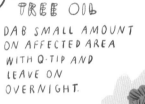

LEMON JUICE
DILUTE WITH WATER, THEN APPLY FOR 20 MINUTES AND RINSE OFF.

GARLIC
DILUTE GARLIC JUICE WITH WATER AND LEAVE ON FOR A FEW MINUTES.

ALOE VERA
APPLY AND LEAVE ON OVERNIGHT.

TOOTHPASTE
DAB TOOTHPASTE (NOT GEL KIND) ON TOP OF ZIT AND LEAVE ON OVERNIGHT.

BAKING SODA
MIX WITH WATER TO CREATE PASTE. USE AS FACIAL. LEAVE ON FOR 15 MINUTES BEFORE RINSING OFF.

EASY HOME REMEDIES FOR TREATING DRY SKIN IN THE WINTER

FOR DRY FACE

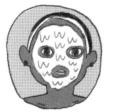

YOU CAN USE COMMON KITCHEN ITEMS TO CREATE YOUR OWN DIY FACIAL MASK. APPLY FOR 15 MINUTES AND RINSE OFF.

 GREEK YOGURT (PLAIN, NO SUGAR)

AVOCADO (MASH INTO PASTE)

PAPAYA + BANANA (MASH TOGETHER INTO A PASTE)

FOR DRY HANDS

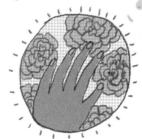

APPLY ANY OF THE FOLLOWING DIRECTLY ONTO YOUR HANDS:

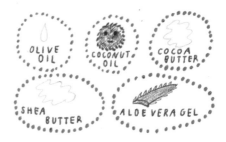

OLIVE OIL

COCONUT OIL

COCOA BUTTER

SHEA BUTTER

ALOE VERA GEL

FOR DRY FEET

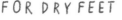

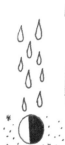

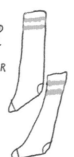

BEFORE GOING TO BED, APPLY HYDROGENATED VEGETABLE OIL TO YOUR FEET AND THEN WEAR THICK COTTON SOCKS. REPEAT FOR SEVERAL NIGHTS.

FOR DRY BODY

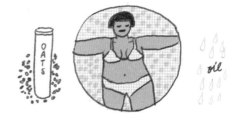

GRIND 1 CUP OF UNCOOKED OATMEAL INTO A FINE POWDER WITH A FOOD PROCESSOR. ADD OATMEAL TO BATH WHILE WATER IS RUNNING. SOAK YOURSELF AND ENJOY!

AFTER BATHING (MAKE SURE WATER IS NOT TOO HOT), APPLY GRAPE-SEED OIL LIBERALLY ONTO YOUR SKIN TO HELP RETAIN MOISTURE.

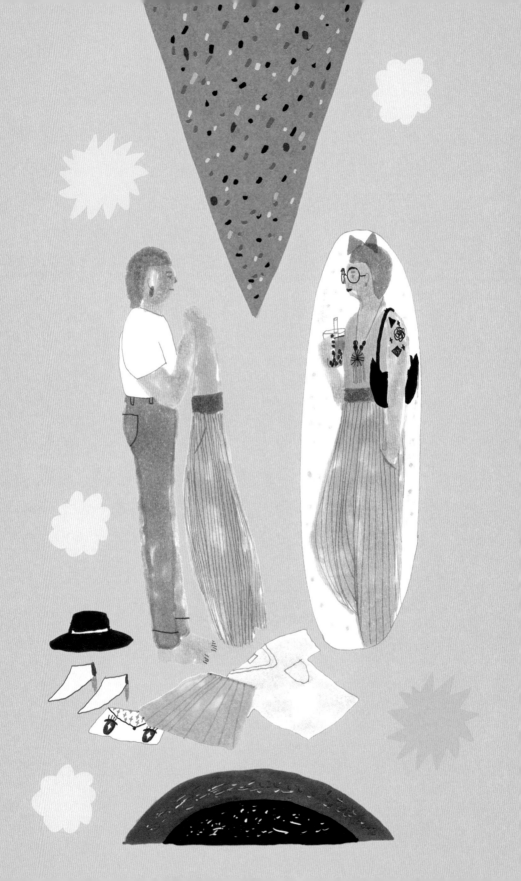

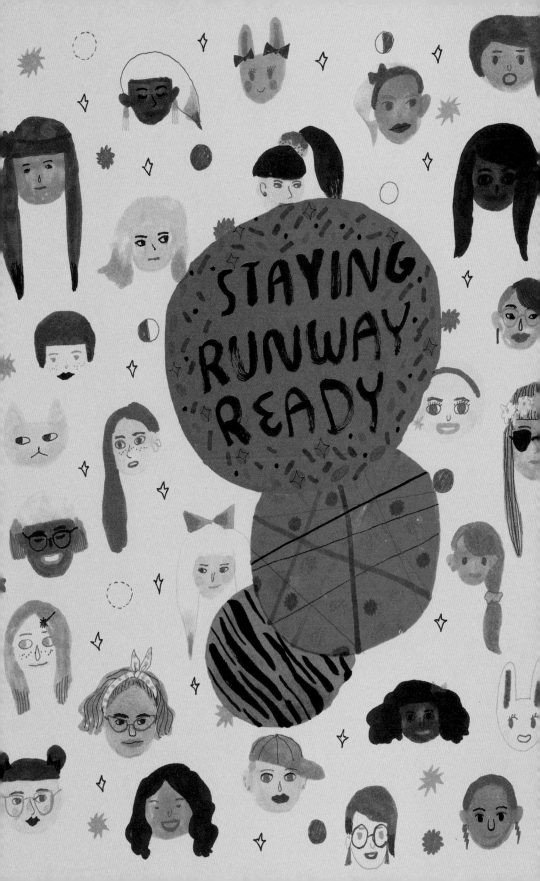

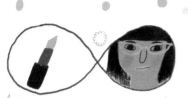

8 DOUBLE-DUTY MAKEUP TOOLS

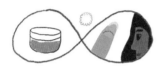

✧ LIPSTICK AS BLUSH ✧
(BEST WITH SOFT SHADES OF PINK)
DOT CHEEKBONES WITH LIPSTICK AND
BLEND IN SMALL, CIRCULAR MOTIONS.

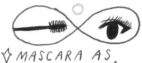

✧ CONCEALER AS
EYE SHADOW PRIMER ✧
DAB SMALL AMOUNT OVER
CLOSED EYELIDS WITH FINGERTIPS,
THEN APPLY EYE SHADOW OVER
LAYER.

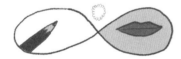

✧ LIP BALM AS CUTICLE
CREAM OR FOR TAMING
FLYAWAY HAIR ✧

✧ MASCARA AS
EYELINER ✧

CAREFULLY APPLY BRUSH ALONG
LASH LINE (NOT WATER LINE) TO
CREATE A SMUDGY LINE, OR USE
A SMALL BRUSH TO APPLY MASCARA
DIRECTLY ONTO EYELIDS AS
EYELINER.

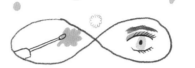

✧ SOFT LIGHT BROWN
EYELINER PENCIL AS
LIP LINER OR BROW
DEFINER ✧

✧ EYE SHADOW AS
EYELINER OR
BROW SHADER ✧
DAMPEN FINE-TIPPED MAKEUP
BRUSH WITH WATER, THEN
DIP INTO EYE SHADOW AND
PAINT ALONG LASH LINE.
OR USE BROWN EYE SHADOW
TO SHADE IN YOUR EYEBROWS.

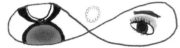

✧ BRONZER AS
EYE SHADOW ✧

✧ CREAM BLUSH AS
LIP GLOSS ✧

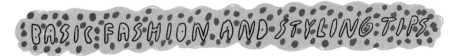

◆ WEAR CLOTHES THAT EMPHASIZE AND AMPLIFY YOUR BEST FEATURES. THEY SHOULD BE FLATTERING SPECIFICALLY TO YOUR BODY TYPE, AND ALSO TRULY REFLECT YOUR UNIQUE PERSONALITY/STYLE. EVERYONE IS DIFFERENT! IF SOMETHING DOESN'T FIT PERFECTLY, CONSIDER GETTING IT TAILORED. IT MAKES A HUGE DIFFERENCE.

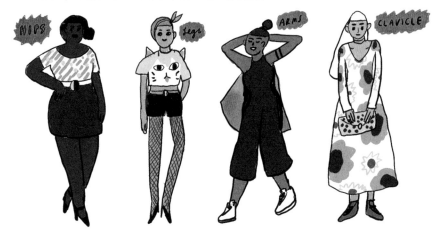

◆ FIND OUT WHICH COLORS ARE THE MOST FLATTERING FOR YOUR SKIN TONE / HAIR. THE EASIEST WAY IS TO CHECK IF YOU HAVE WARM OR COOL UNDERTONES.

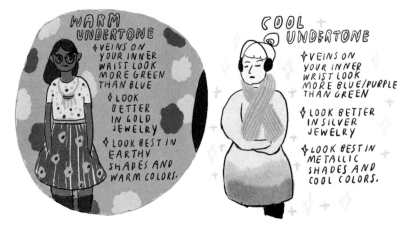

WARM UNDERTONE

◆ VEINS ON YOUR INNER WRIST LOOK MORE GREEN THAN BLUE

◆ LOOK BETTER IN GOLD JEWELRY

◆ LOOK BEST IN EARTHY SHADES AND WARM COLORS.

COOL UNDERTONE

◆ VEINS ON YOUR INNER WRIST LOOK MORE BLUE/PURPLE THAN GREEN

◆ LOOK BETTER IN SILVER JEWELRY

◆ LOOK BEST IN METALLIC SHADES AND COOL COLORS.

◆ TIP ◆ FLATTERING COLORS SHOULD MAKE YOU LOOK MORE VIBRANT, WHEREAS UNFLATTERING COLORS WILL MAKE YOU LOOK WASHED OUT.

◆ EXPERIMENT WITH DIFFERENT CUTS, STYLES, AND SILHOUETTES. IF YOU FIND YOURSELF BUYING/ WEARING THE SAME STYLE, TRY SOMETHING DIFFERENT!

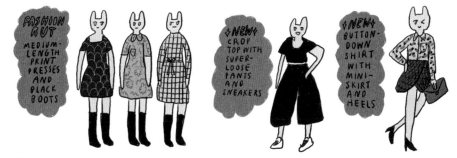

FASHION RUT MEDIUM-LENGTH PRINT DRESSES AND BLACK BOOTS

✦NEW✦ CROP TOP WITH SUPER-LOOSE PANTS AND SNEAKERS

✦NEW✦ BUTTON-DOWN SHIRT WITH MINI-SKIRT AND HEELS

◆ WHO ARE YOUR FASHION ICONS? WHAT KIND OF AESTHETIC STYLES ARE YOU DRAWN TO? WHAT STYLES EXCITE YOU / INTIMIDATE YOU? TAKE NOTE AND TAKE RISKS!

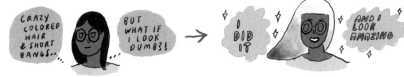

CRAZY COLORED HAIR & SHORT BANGS...

BUT WHAT IF I LOOK DUMB?!

→

I DID IT

AND I LOOK AMAZING

◆ DON'T BE A SLAVE TO TRENDS. ONLY FOLLOW A FASHION TREND IF YOU LOVE IT AND IT IS SUPER-FLATTERING TO YOU!

◆ IN CONCLUSION ◆ WEAR WHAT MAKES YOU FEEL MOST BEAUTIFUL AND UNABASHEDLY YOU. DISCOVERING, CREATING, AND LIVING YOUR OWN UNIQUE FASHION STYLE IS A LIFELONG JOURNEY!

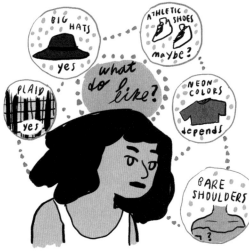

BIG HATS yes

ATHLETIC SHOES maybe?

what do I like?

NEON COLORS depends

PLAID yes

BARE SHOULDERS ?

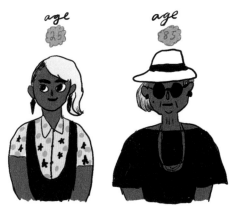

age 25

age 85

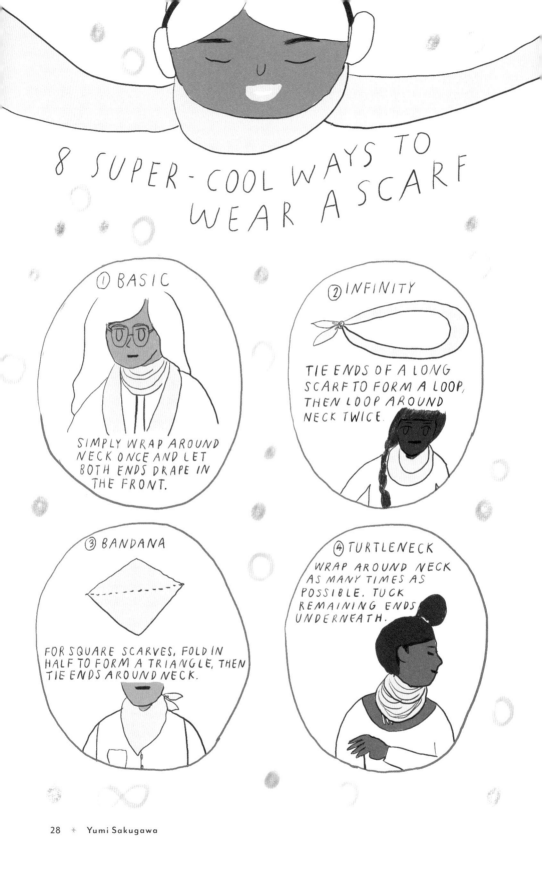

8 SUPER-COOL WAYS TO WEAR A SCARF

① BASIC

SIMPLY WRAP AROUND NECK ONCE AND LET BOTH ENDS DRAPE IN THE FRONT.

② INFINITY

TIE ENDS OF A LONG SCARF TO FORM A LOOP, THEN LOOP AROUND NECK TWICE.

③ BANDANA

FOR SQUARE SCARVES, FOLD IN HALF TO FORM A TRIANGLE, THEN TIE ENDS AROUND NECK.

④ TURTLENECK

WRAP AROUND NECK AS MANY TIMES AS POSSIBLE. TUCK REMAINING ENDS UNDERNEATH.

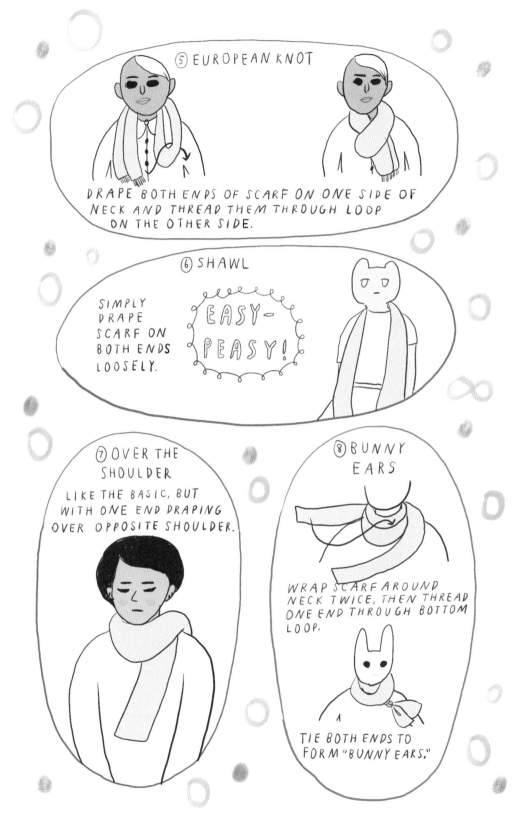

⑤ EUROPEAN KNOT

DRAPE BOTH ENDS OF SCARF ON ONE SIDE OF NECK AND THREAD THEM THROUGH LOOP ON THE OTHER SIDE.

⑥ SHAWL

SIMPLY DRAPE SCARF ON BOTH ENDS LOOSELY.

EASY-PEASY!

⑦ OVER THE SHOULDER

LIKE THE BASIC, BUT WITH ONE END DRAPING OVER OPPOSITE SHOULDER.

⑧ BUNNY EARS

WRAP SCARF AROUND NECK TWICE, THEN THREAD ONE END THROUGH BOTTOM LOOP.

TIE BOTH ENDS TO FORM "BUNNY EARS."

wardrobe makeover: cheap ways to add pizzazz to your existing clothes

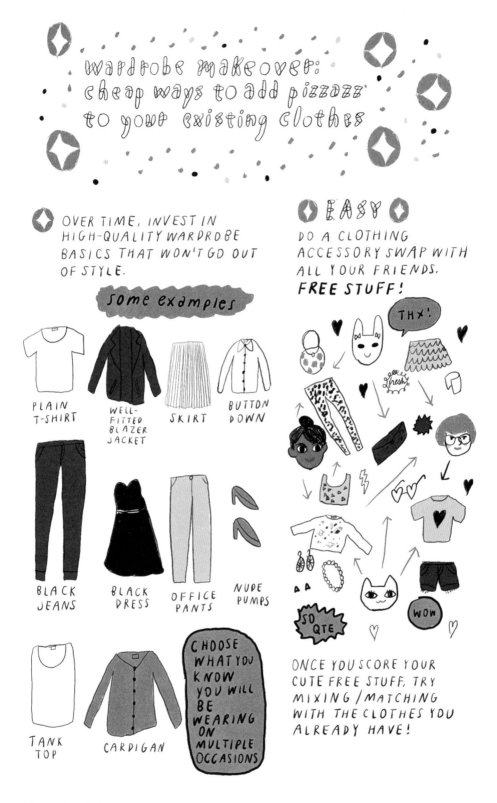

OVER TIME, INVEST IN HIGH-QUALITY WARDROBE BASICS THAT WON'T GO OUT OF STYLE.

some examples

PLAIN T-SHIRT

WELL-FITTED BLAZER JACKET

SKIRT

BUTTON DOWN

BLACK JEANS

BLACK DRESS

OFFICE PANTS

NUDE PUMPS

TANK TOP

CARDIGAN

CHOOSE WHAT YOU KNOW YOU WILL BE WEARING ON MULTIPLE OCCASIONS

EASY

DO A CLOTHING ACCESSORY SWAP WITH ALL YOUR FRIENDS. **FREE STUFF!**

THX!

fresh!

SO QTE

WOW

ONCE YOU SCORE YOUR CUTE FREE STUFF, TRY MIXING / MATCHING WITH THE CLOTHES YOU ALREADY HAVE!

KEEP A LOOKOUT FOR EYE-CATCHING
JEWELRY AND ACCESSORIES IN UNEXPECTED
PLACES (THRIFT STORES, CONSIGNMENT STORES,
FLEA MARKETS, GARAGE SALES, YARD SALES,
FREE BOXES, ONLINE SALES, ETC.). ONE
STATEMENT JEWELRY OR ACCESSORY PIECE
CAN COMPLETELY TRANSFORM A NEUTRAL
OUTFIT, ESPECIALLY IF PAIRED WITH A
BOLD LIPSTICK SHADE OR EYE MAKEUP.

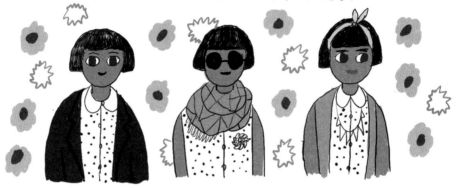

FURTHER ENHANCE / UPGRADE YOUR WARDROBE BY
ALTERING / MODIFYING WHAT YOU ALREADY HAVE,
OR MAKING YOUR OWN ACCESSORIES. BIG BONUS
IF YOU KNOW HOW TO SEW. (OR, TAKE KEY
WARDROBE ITEMS TO A TAILOR SO THEY LOOK
BRAND-NEW ON YOU.)

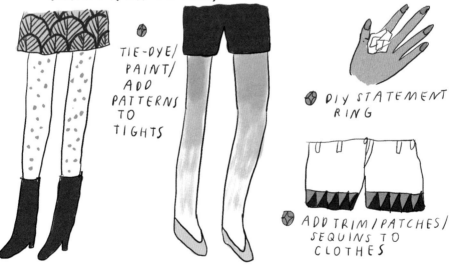

TIE-DYE/
PAINT/
ADD
PATTERNS
TO
TIGHTS

DIY STATEMENT
RING

ADD TRIM / PATCHES /
SEQUINS TO
CLOTHES

GET THE MOST MILEAGE OUT OF YOUR WARDROBE BY MIXING AND MATCHING ITEMS AND ACCESSORIES.

ALSO EXPERIMENT WITH DIFFERENT HAIRSTYLES, MAKEUP COLOR PALETTES, EVEN MANICURE COLORS. MOST IMPORTANT, HAVE FUN AND WEAR WHAT MAKES YOU HAPPY!

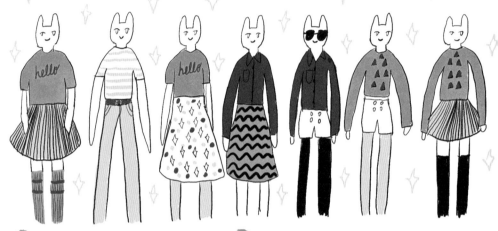

COLLECT FASHION INSPIRATION THROUGH WEBSITES AND MAGAZINES TO GET A SENSE OF WHAT YOU VISUALLY GRAVITATE TOWARD. PEOPLE-WATCH/ WINDOW-SHOP. DAYDREAM AMAZING OUTFITS AND HOW YOU FEEL WEARING THEM.

LAST... THERE IS NOTHING WRONG WITH HAVING THE SAME SIGNATURE LOOK EVERY DAY, WHICH IS ALSO A FASHION STATEMENT IN ITSELF.

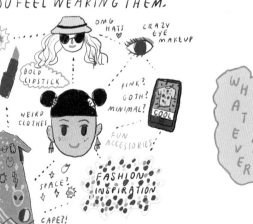

OMG HATS ♥

CRAZY EYE MAKEUP

BOLD LIPSTICK

PINK? GOTH? MINIMAL!

COOL

WEIRD CLOTHES

FUN ACCESSORIES!

SPACE?

FASHION INSPIRATION

CAPE?!

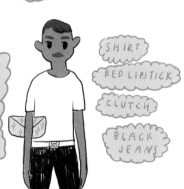

MON – FRI

WHATEVER

SHIRT

RED LIPSTICK

CLUTCH

BLACK JEANS

HOW TO REMOVE SCUFF MARKS FROM SHOES

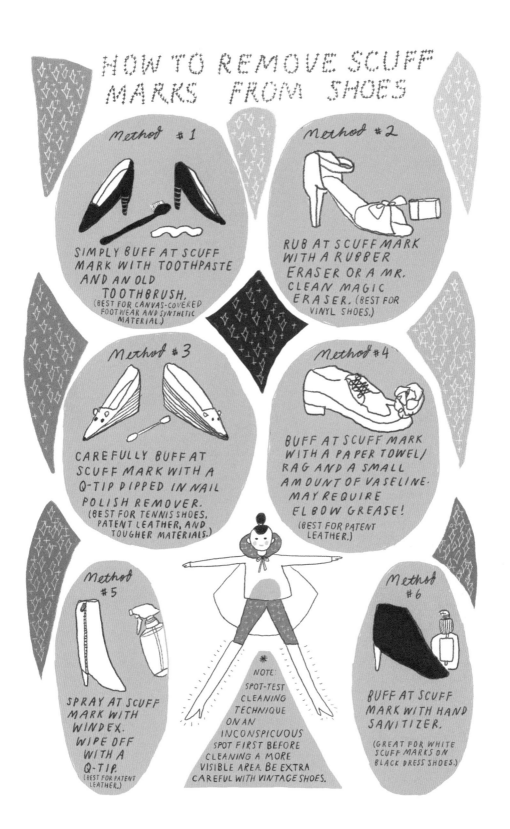

Method #1

SIMPLY BUFF AT SCUFF MARK WITH TOOTHPASTE AND AN OLD TOOTHBRUSH. (BEST FOR CANVAS-COVERED FOOTWEAR AND SYNTHETIC MATERIAL.)

Method #2

RUB AT SCUFF MARK WITH A RUBBER ERASER OR A MR. CLEAN MAGIC ERASER. (BEST FOR VINYL SHOES.)

Method #3

CAREFULLY BUFF AT SCUFF MARK WITH A Q-TIP DIPPED IN NAIL POLISH REMOVER. (BEST FOR TENNIS SHOES, PATENT LEATHER, AND TOUGHER MATERIALS.)

Method #4

BUFF AT SCUFF MARK WITH A PAPER TOWEL/ RAG AND A SMALL AMOUNT OF VASELINE. MAY REQUIRE ELBOW GREASE! (BEST FOR PATENT LEATHER.)

Method #5

SPRAY AT SCUFF MARK WITH WINDEX. WIPE OFF WITH A Q-TIP. (BEST FOR PATENT LEATHER.)

NOTE: SPOT-TEST CLEANING TECHNIQUE ON AN INCONSPICUOUS SPOT FIRST BEFORE CLEANING A MORE VISIBLE AREA. BE EXTRA CAREFUL WITH VINTAGE SHOES.

Method #6

BUFF AT SCUFF MARK WITH HAND SANITIZER. (GREAT FOR WHITE SCUFF MARKS ON BLACK DRESS SHOES.)

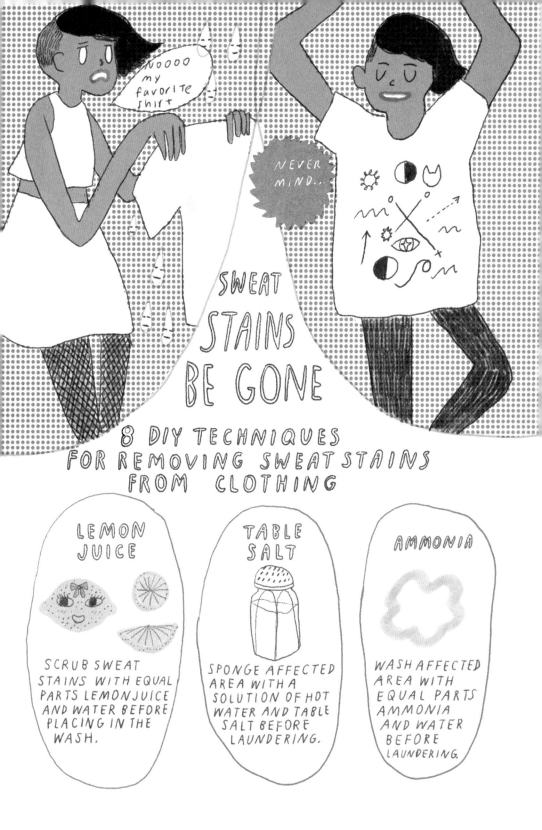

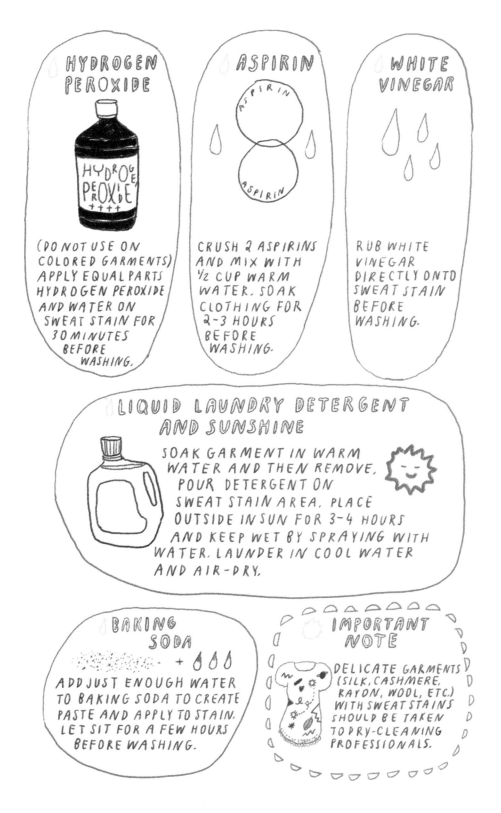

HYDROGEN PEROXIDE

(DO NOT USE ON COLORED GARMENTS) APPLY EQUAL PARTS HYDROGEN PEROXIDE AND WATER ON SWEAT STAIN FOR 30 MINUTES BEFORE WASHING.

ASPIRIN

CRUSH 2 ASPIRINS AND MIX WITH ½ CUP WARM WATER. SOAK CLOTHING FOR 2-3 HOURS BEFORE WASHING.

ASPIRIN

ASPIRIN

WHITE VINEGAR

RUB WHITE VINEGAR DIRECTLY ONTO SWEAT STAIN BEFORE WASHING.

LIQUID LAUNDRY DETERGENT AND SUNSHINE

SOAK GARMENT IN WARM WATER AND THEN REMOVE. POUR DETERGENT ON SWEAT STAIN AREA. PLACE OUTSIDE IN SUN FOR 3-4 HOURS AND KEEP WET BY SPRAYING WITH WATER. LAUNDER IN COOL WATER AND AIR-DRY.

BAKING SODA

ADD JUST ENOUGH WATER TO BAKING SODA TO CREATE PASTE AND APPLY TO STAIN. LET SIT FOR A FEW HOURS BEFORE WASHING.

IMPORTANT NOTE

DELICATE GARMENTS (SILK, CASHMERE, RAYON, WOOL, ETC.) WITH SWEAT STAINS SHOULD BE TAKEN TO DRY-CLEANING PROFESSIONALS.

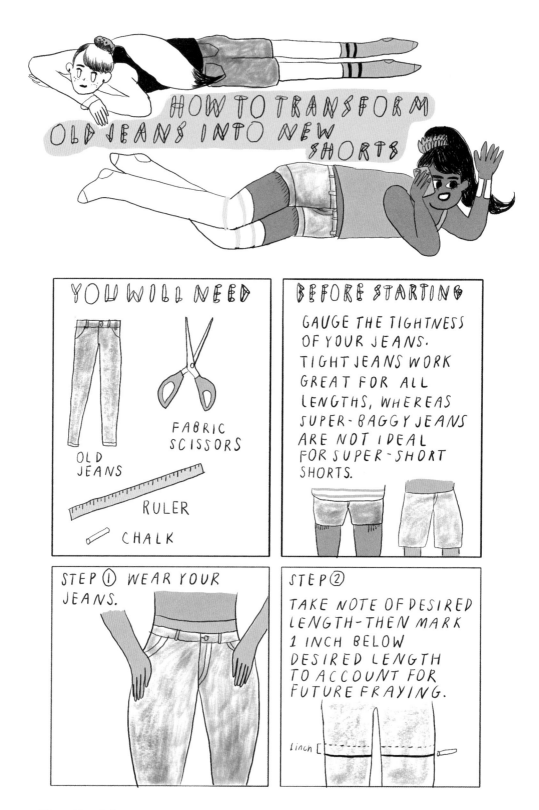

HOW TO TRANSFORM OLD JEANS INTO NEW SHORTS

YOU WILL NEED

OLD JEANS

FABRIC SCISSORS

RULER

CHALK

BEFORE STARTING

GAUGE THE TIGHTNESS OF YOUR JEANS. TIGHT JEANS WORK GREAT FOR ALL LENGTHS, WHEREAS SUPER-BAGGY JEANS ARE NOT IDEAL FOR SUPER-SHORT SHORTS.

STEP ① WEAR YOUR JEANS.

STEP ②

TAKE NOTE OF DESIRED LENGTH—THEN MARK 1 INCH BELOW DESIRED LENGTH TO ACCOUNT FOR FUTURE FRAYING.

1 inch

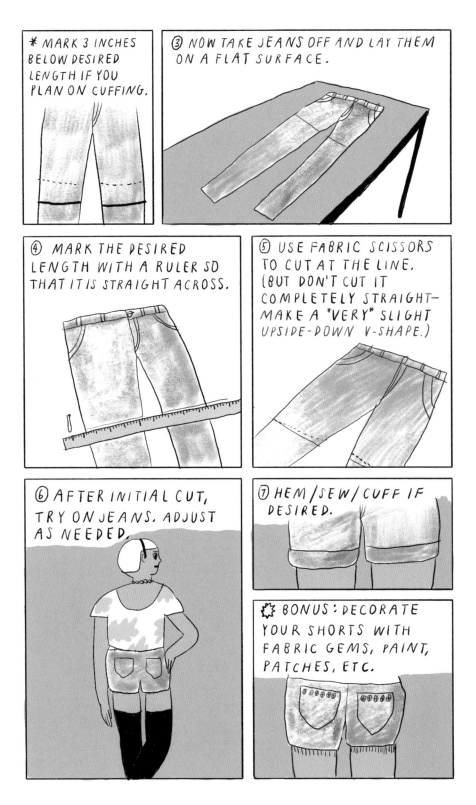

✱ MARK 3 INCHES BELOW DESIRED LENGTH IF YOU PLAN ON CUFFING.

③ NOW TAKE JEANS OFF AND LAY THEM ON A FLAT SURFACE.

④ MARK THE DESIRED LENGTH WITH A RULER SO THAT IT IS STRAIGHT ACROSS.

⑤ USE FABRIC SCISSORS TO CUT AT THE LINE. (BUT DON'T CUT IT COMPLETELY STRAIGHT— MAKE A *VERY* SLIGHT UPSIDE-DOWN V-SHAPE.)

⑥ AFTER INITIAL CUT, TRY ON JEANS. ADJUST AS NEEDED.

⑦ HEM/SEW/CUFF IF DESIRED.

✿ BONUS: DECORATE YOUR SHORTS WITH FABRIC GEMS, PAINT, PATCHES, ETC.

HOW TO REMOVE WRINKLES FROM CLOTHING W/O IRONING

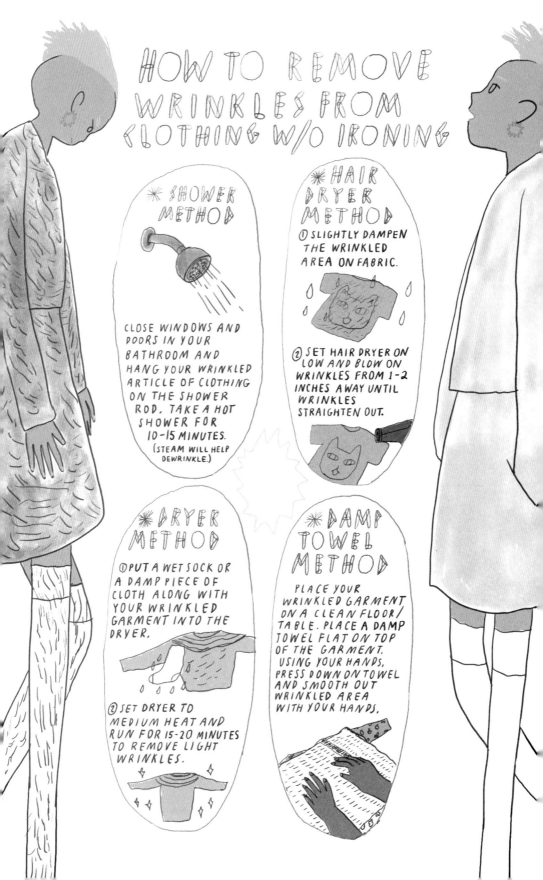

* SHOWER METHOD

CLOSE WINDOWS AND DOORS IN YOUR BATHROOM AND HANG YOUR WRINKLED ARTICLE OF CLOTHING ON THE SHOWER ROD. TAKE A HOT SHOWER FOR 10-15 MINUTES. (STEAM WILL HELP DEWRINKLE.)

* HAIR DRYER METHOD

① SLIGHTLY DAMPEN THE WRINKLED AREA ON FABRIC.

② SET HAIR DRYER ON LOW AND BLOW ON WRINKLES FROM 1-2 INCHES AWAY UNTIL WRINKLES STRAIGHTEN OUT.

* DRYER METHOD

① PUT A WET SOCK OR A DAMP PIECE OF CLOTH ALONG WITH YOUR WRINKLED GARMENT INTO THE DRYER.

② SET DRYER TO MEDIUM HEAT AND RUN FOR 15-20 MINUTES TO REMOVE LIGHT WRINKLES.

* DAMP TOWEL METHOD

PLACE YOUR WRINKLED GARMENT ON A CLEAN FLOOR/ TABLE. PLACE A DAMP TOWEL FLAT ON TOP OF THE GARMENT. USING YOUR HANDS, PRESS DOWN ON TOWEL AND SMOOTH OUT WRINKLED AREA WITH YOUR HANDS.

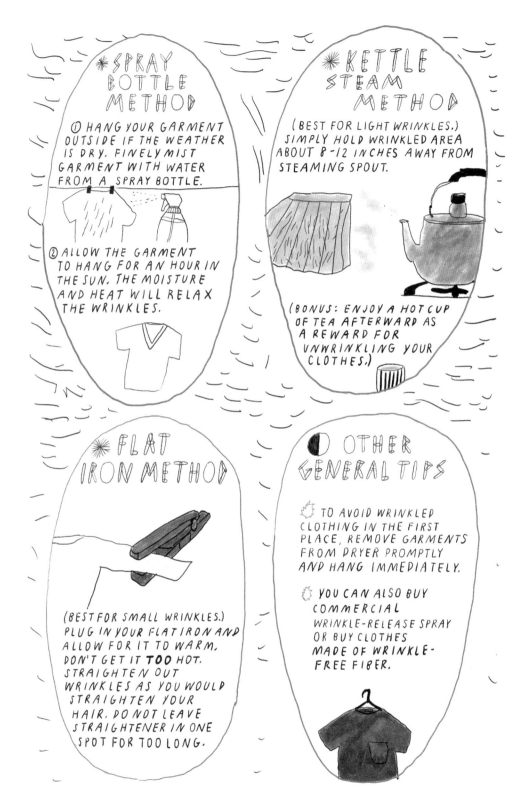

*SPRAY BOTTLE METHOD

① HANG YOUR GARMENT OUTSIDE IF THE WEATHER IS DRY. FINELY MIST GARMENT WITH WATER FROM A SPRAY BOTTLE.

② ALLOW THE GARMENT TO HANG FOR AN HOUR IN THE SUN. THE MOISTURE AND HEAT WILL RELAX THE WRINKLES.

*KETTLE STEAM METHOD

(BEST FOR LIGHT WRINKLES.) SIMPLY HOLD WRINKLED AREA ABOUT 8-12 INCHES AWAY FROM STEAMING SPOUT.

(BONUS: ENJOY A HOT CUP OF TEA AFTERWARD AS A REWARD FOR UNWRINKLING YOUR CLOTHES.)

*FLAT IRON METHOD

(BEST FOR SMALL WRINKLES.) PLUG IN YOUR FLAT IRON AND ALLOW FOR IT TO WARM. DON'T GET IT **TOO** HOT. STRAIGHTEN OUT WRINKLES AS YOU WOULD STRAIGHTEN YOUR HAIR. DO NOT LEAVE STRAIGHTENER IN ONE SPOT FOR TOO LONG.

◑ OTHER GENERAL TIPS

✦ TO AVOID WRINKLED CLOTHING IN THE FIRST PLACE, REMOVE GARMENTS FROM DRYER PROMPTLY AND HANG IMMEDIATELY.

✦ YOU CAN ALSO BUY COMMERCIAL WRINKLE-RELEASE SPRAY OR BUY CLOTHES MADE OF WRINKLE-FREE FIBER.

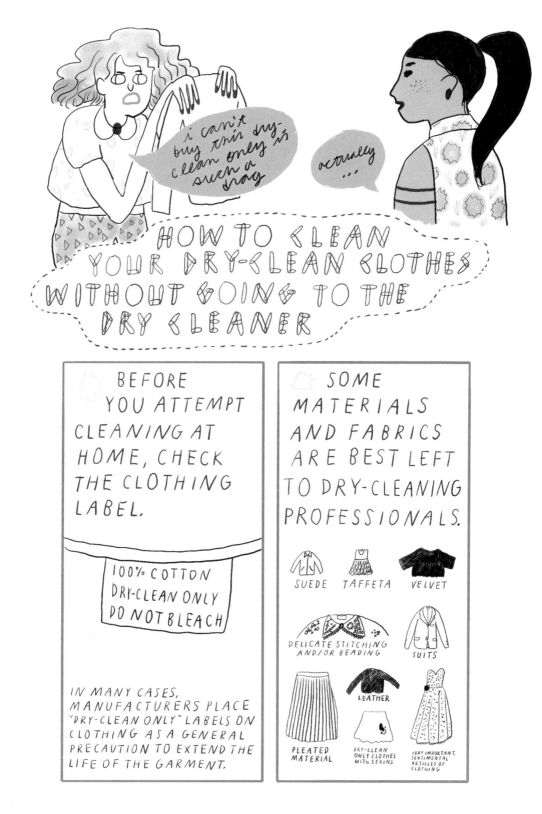

BEFORE WASHING DRY-CLEAN ONLY CLOTHING AT HOME, CHECK FABRIC (ESPECIALLY RED OR DEEP-COLORED FABRICS) FOR COLORFASTEDNESS. WET AN INCONSPICUOUS AREA OF YOUR CLOTHING ITEM WITH A FEW DROPS OF WATER AND PRESS A WHITE COTTON SWAB AGAINST THE DAMP AREA. IF THE COLOR BLEEDS, CLOTHING ITEM SHOULD BE TAKEN TO DRY CLEANERS ONLY.

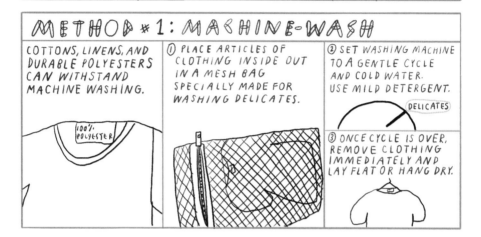

METHOD #1: MACHINE-WASH

COTTONS, LINENS, AND DURABLE POLYESTERS CAN WITHSTAND MACHINE WASHING.

① PLACE ARTICLES OF CLOTHING INSIDE OUT IN A MESH BAG SPECIALLY MADE FOR WASHING DELICATES.

② SET WASHING MACHINE TO A GENTLE CYCLE AND COLD WATER. USE MILD DETERGENT.

③ ONCE CYCLE IS OVER, REMOVE CLOTHING IMMEDIATELY AND LAY FLAT OR HANG DRY.

METHOD #2: HAND-WASH

WOOL, SILK, AND COTTON CAN WITHSTAND HAND-WASHING.

① FILL A SINK OR BUCKET WITH COLD WATER AND ADD A MILD DETERGENT. MIX A LITTLE TO CREATE FOAM. (FOR WOOL PRODUCTS, USE A DETERGENT LIKE WOOLITE.)

② DIP CLOTHING IN AND OUT OF SOAPY WATER UNTIL EVERYTHING IS SOAKED THROUGH. RUB AT SOILED AREAS WITH FINGERTIPS.

③ DRAIN SOAPY WATER AND REFILL WITH COLD WATER AGAIN. DIP AND REDIP CLOTHING IN WATER UNTIL ALL THE SOAP IS GONE. REFILL BASIN/BUCKET WITH WATER AGAIN IF NEEDED.

④ LAY CLOTHING ON CLEAN WHITE TOWEL AND PUSH (DO NOT TWIST) WATER OUT. PLACE ANOTHER TOWEL ON TOP AND ROLL TOWEL UP WHILE SQUEEZING GENTLY. REPEAT 3-5 TIMES. RESHAPE GARMENT AND LAY FLAT ON ANOTHER CLEAN DRY TOWEL UNTIL DRY. KEEP AWAY FROM SUNLIGHT/HEAT.

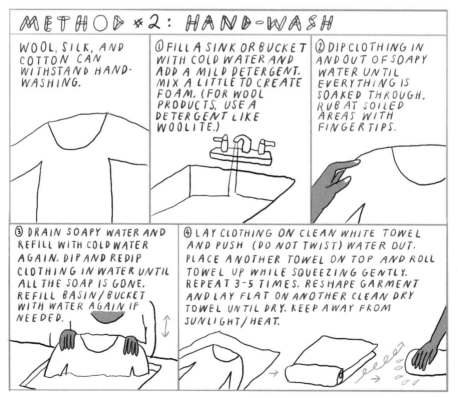

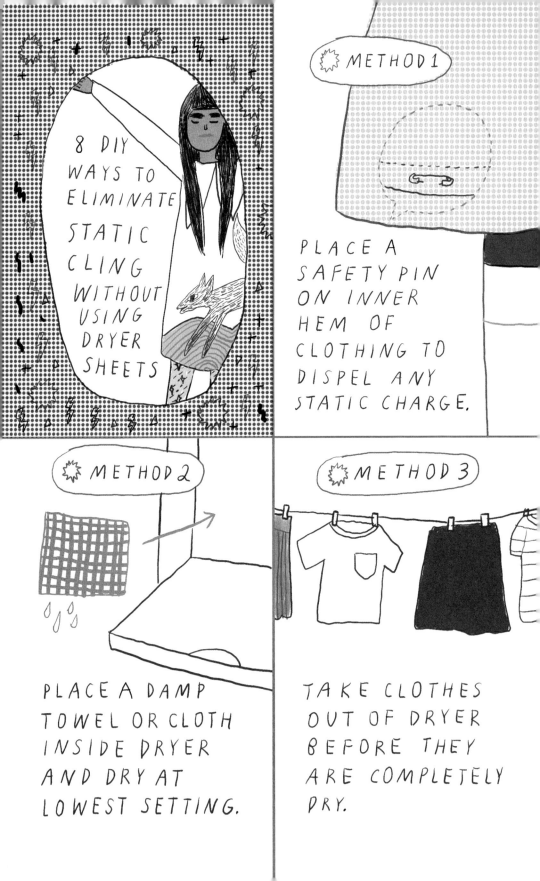

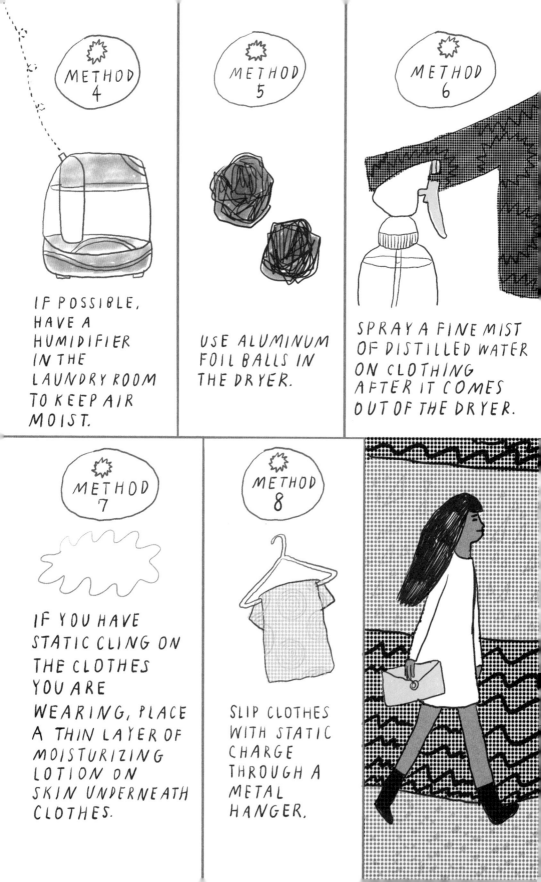

METHOD 4

IF POSSIBLE, HAVE A HUMIDIFIER IN THE LAUNDRY ROOM TO KEEP AIR MOIST.

METHOD 5

USE ALUMINUM FOIL BALLS IN THE DRYER.

METHOD 6

SPRAY A FINE MIST OF DISTILLED WATER ON CLOTHING AFTER IT COMES OUT OF THE DRYER.

METHOD 7

IF YOU HAVE STATIC CLING ON THE CLOTHES YOU ARE WEARING, PLACE A THIN LAYER OF MOISTURIZING LOTION ON SKIN UNDERNEATH CLOTHES.

METHOD 8

SLIP CLOTHES WITH STATIC CHARGE THROUGH A METAL HANGER.

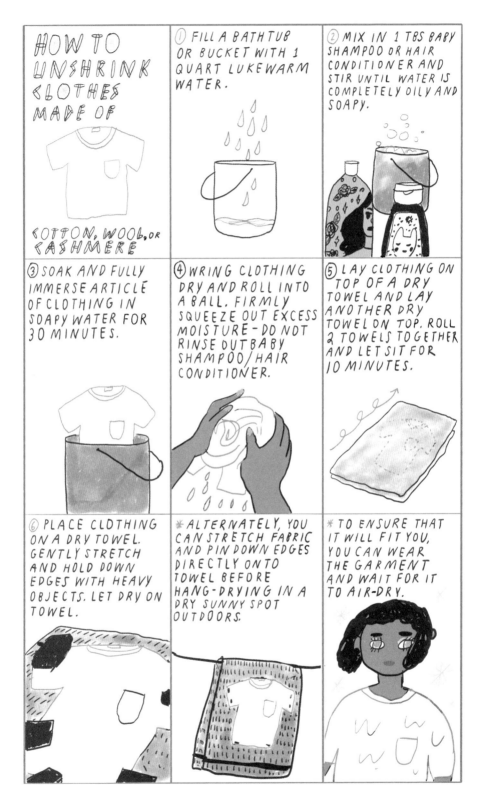

HOW TO UNSHRINK CLOTHES MADE OF

COTTON, WOOL, OR CASHMERE

1. FILL A BATHTUB OR BUCKET WITH 1 QUART LUKEWARM WATER.

2. MIX IN 1 TBS BABY SHAMPOO OR HAIR CONDITIONER AND STIR UNTIL WATER IS COMPLETELY OILY AND SOAPY.

3. SOAK AND FULLY IMMERSE ARTICLE OF CLOTHING IN SOAPY WATER FOR 30 MINUTES.

4. WRING CLOTHING DRY AND ROLL INTO A BALL. FIRMLY SQUEEZE OUT EXCESS MOISTURE — DO NOT RINSE OUT BABY SHAMPOO/HAIR CONDITIONER.

5. LAY CLOTHING ON TOP OF A DRY TOWEL AND LAY ANOTHER DRY TOWEL ON TOP. ROLL 2 TOWELS TOGETHER AND LET SIT FOR 10 MINUTES.

6. PLACE CLOTHING ON A DRY TOWEL. GENTLY STRETCH AND HOLD DOWN EDGES WITH HEAVY OBJECTS. LET DRY ON TOWEL.

* ALTERNATELY, YOU CAN STRETCH FABRIC AND PIN DOWN EDGES DIRECTLY ONTO TOWEL BEFORE HANG-DRYING IN A DRY SUNNY SPOT OUTDOORS.

* TO ENSURE THAT IT WILL FIT YOU, YOU CAN WEAR THE GARMENT AND WAIT FOR IT TO AIR-DRY.

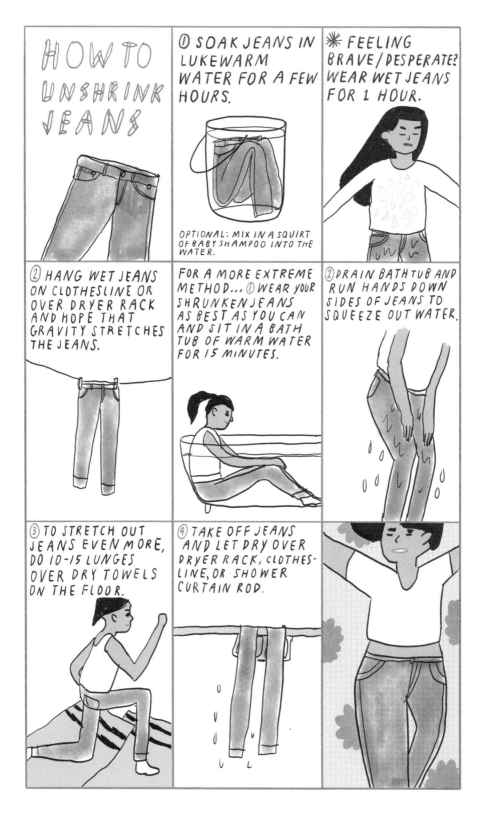

HOW TO UNSHRINK JEANS

① SOAK JEANS IN LUKEWARM WATER FOR A FEW HOURS.

OPTIONAL: MIX IN A SQUIRT OF BABY SHAMPOO INTO THE WATER.

✳ FEELING BRAVE / DESPERATE? WEAR WET JEANS FOR 1 HOUR.

② HANG WET JEANS ON CLOTHESLINE OR OVER DRYER RACK AND HOPE THAT GRAVITY STRETCHES THE JEANS.

FOR A MORE EXTREME METHOD... ① WEAR YOUR SHRUNKEN JEANS AS BEST AS YOU CAN AND SIT IN A BATH TUB OF WARM WATER FOR 15 MINUTES.

② DRAIN BATH TUB AND RUN HANDS DOWN SIDES OF JEANS TO SQUEEZE OUT WATER.

③ TO STRETCH OUT JEANS EVEN MORE, DO 10-15 LUNGES OVER DRY TOWELS ON THE FLOOR.

④ TAKE OFF JEANS AND LET DRY OVER DRYER RACK, CLOTHES-LINE, OR SHOWER CURTAIN ROD.

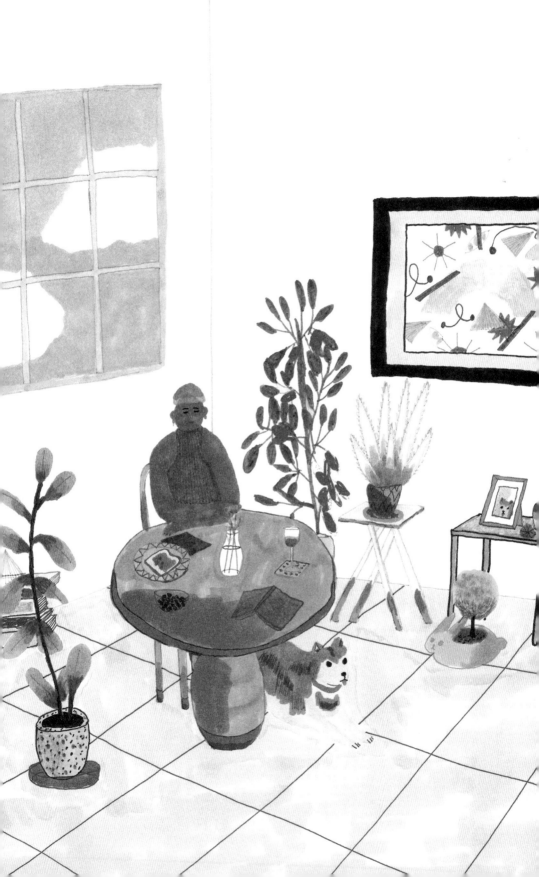

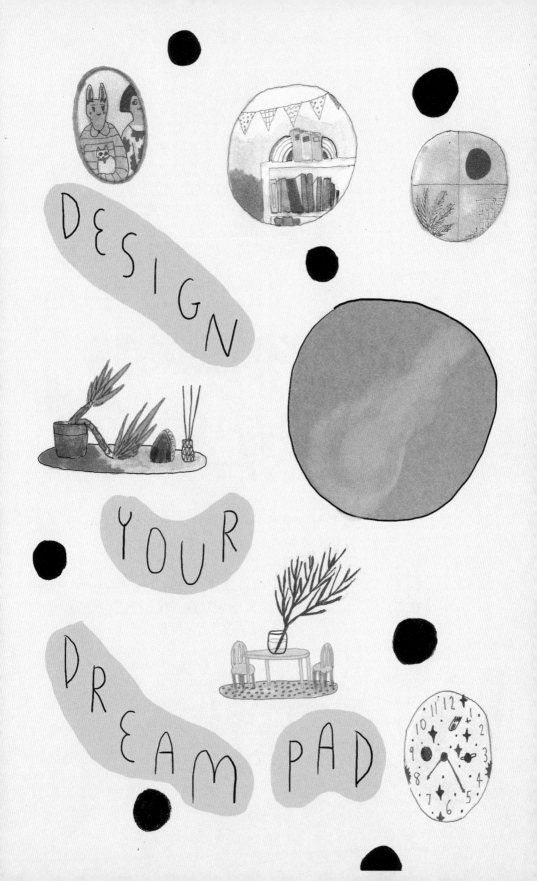

DESIGN

YOUR

DREAM PAD

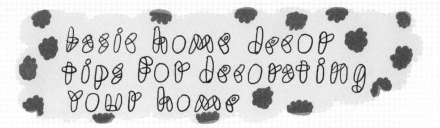

✦ CHOOSE A FOCAL POINT IN EACH ROOM AS A VISUAL ANCHOR TO DECORATE AROUND. FOR EXAMPLE, IF YOU HAVE A REALLY AWESOME COUCH IN YOUR LIVING ROOM, DECORATE AROUND IT! PLACE A STRIKING PAINTING ABOVE IT, PLANTS ON EITHER SIDE OF IT, ETC.

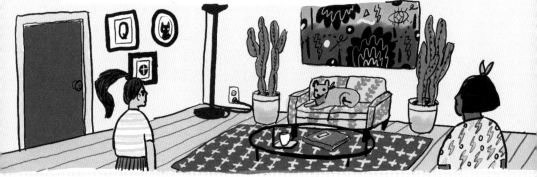

✦ FOR LIVING ROOM AREA RUGS, ALL FOUR LEGS OF THE SOFA AND CHAIRS IN A FURNITURE GROUPING SHOULD FIT ON TOP OF THE RUG, OR AT LEAST THE TWO FRONT LEGS OF THE SOFA SHOULD FIT ON TOP OF THE RUG. IF THE RUG SIZE IS TOO SMALL, EVERYTHING WILL LOOK OUT OF SCALE.

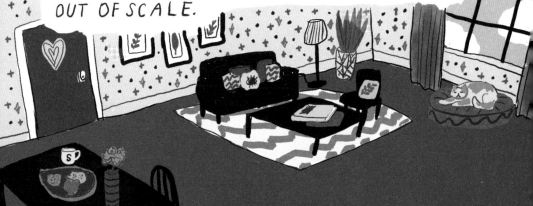

✧ INVEST IN HIGH-QUALITY FURNITURE ITEMS YOU PLAN ON USING FOR A LONG TIME.

✧ GET VISUAL INSPIRATION THROUGH MAGAZINES, BLOGS, OTHER PEOPLE'S HOMES, ETC. TO FIND WHAT COLOR SCHEMES AND INTERIOR DECORATING STYLES EXCITE YOU THE MOST.

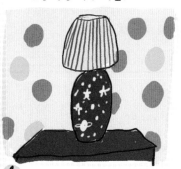

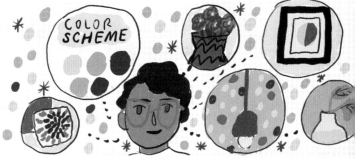

✧ NEGATIVE SPACE IS JUST AS IMPORTANT AS FILLED-IN SPACE! PRIORITIZE IN EACH ROOM WHAT NEEDS TO BE SEEN THE MOST, AND MINIMIZE THE REST.

✧ FLOAT FURNITURE A LITTLE BIT AWAY FROM THE WALLS TO MAKE THE ROOM APPEAR BIGGER.

✧ WHEN HANGING VERY LARGE PRINTS OR ART PIECES, THE CENTER OF THE OBJECT SHOULD BE AT EYE LEVEL.

✧ DECORATE TO YOUR ROOM'S STRENGTHS WHILE MINIMIZING ITS WEAKNESSES. EXAMPLE: IF YOUR LIVING ROOM HAS LOW CEILINGS, INVEST IN LOW COFFEE TABLES AND CHAIRS!

10 WAYS TO MAKE YOUR TINY APARTMENT FEEL LIKE A PALACE

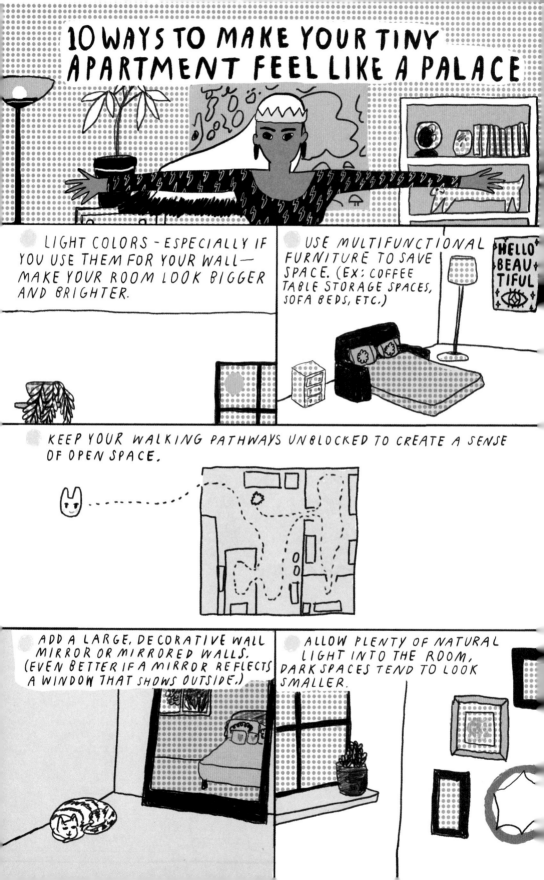

LIGHT COLORS - ESPECIALLY IF YOU USE THEM FOR YOUR WALL— MAKE YOUR ROOM LOOK BIGGER AND BRIGHTER.

USE MULTIFUNCTIONAL FURNITURE TO SAVE SPACE. (EX: COFFEE TABLE STORAGE SPACES, SOFA BEDS, ETC.)

HELLO BEAU TIFUL

KEEP YOUR WALKING PATHWAYS UNBLOCKED TO CREATE A SENSE OF OPEN SPACE.

ADD A LARGE, DECORATIVE WALL MIRROR OR MIRRORED WALLS. (EVEN BETTER IF A MIRROR REFLECTS A WINDOW THAT SHOWS OUTSIDE.)

ALLOW PLENTY OF NATURAL LIGHT INTO THE ROOM, DARK SPACES TEND TO LOOK SMALLER.

HAVE YOUR FURNITURE IN THE SAME COLOR (OR SAME COLOR FAMILY) AS YOUR WALL COLOR.

USE A STRIPED FLOOR RUG (MAKE SURE IT IS PARALLEL TO THE LONGER SIDE OF ROOM).

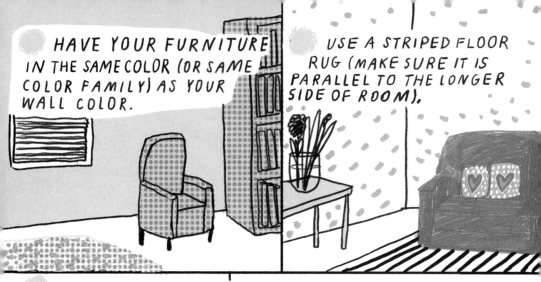

AVOID OVERDECORATING YOUR WALLS. RATHER, HAVE ONE POINT FOR PEOPLE TO FOCUS ON.

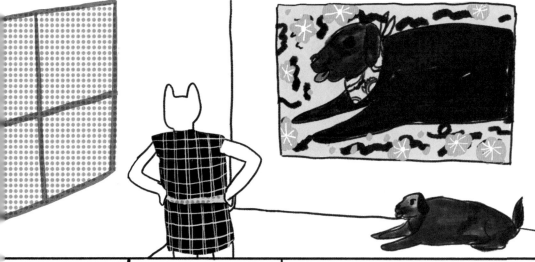

SCALE DOWN THE SIZE OF YOUR FURNITURE. FURNISH WITH SMALL PIECES.

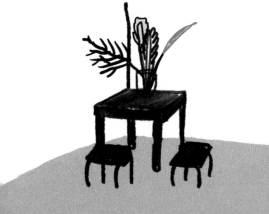

TO ADD MORE ILLUSION OF DEPTH AND SPACE, USE CLEAR THINGS (GLASS TABLETOPS, SHEER DRAPERIES, CLEAR SHOWER CURTAINS, ETC.) INSTEAD OF OPAQUE OBJECTS.

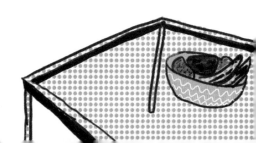

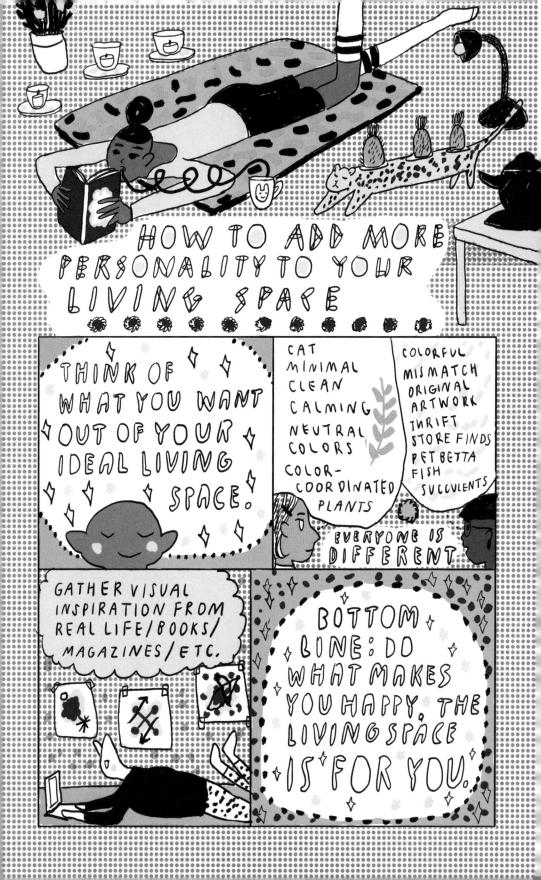

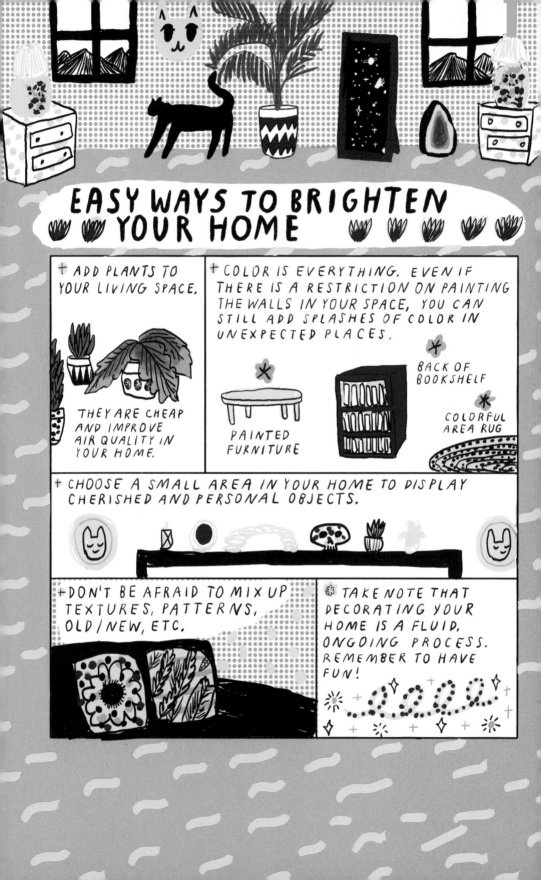

EASY WAYS TO BRIGHTEN YOUR HOME

+ ADD PLANTS TO YOUR LIVING SPACE.

THEY ARE CHEAP AND IMPROVE AIR QUALITY IN YOUR HOME.

+ COLOR IS EVERYTHING. EVEN IF THERE IS A RESTRICTION ON PAINTING THE WALLS IN YOUR SPACE, YOU CAN STILL ADD SPLASHES OF COLOR IN UNEXPECTED PLACES.

PAINTED FURNITURE

BACK OF BOOKSHELF

COLORFUL AREA RUG

+ CHOOSE A SMALL AREA IN YOUR HOME TO DISPLAY CHERISHED AND PERSONAL OBJECTS.

+ DON'T BE AFRAID TO MIX UP TEXTURES, PATTERNS, OLD/NEW, ETC.

❀ TAKE NOTE THAT DECORATING YOUR HOME IS A FLUID, ONGOING PROCESS. REMEMBER TO HAVE FUN!

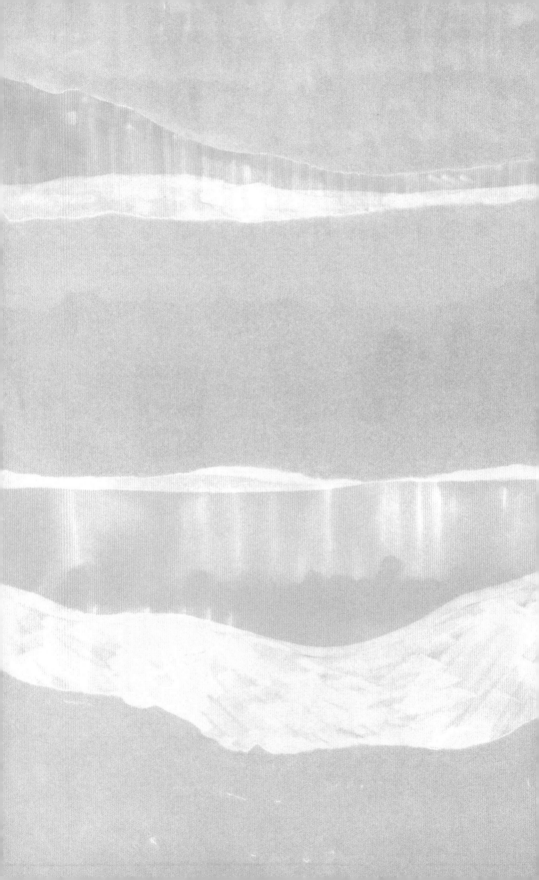

12 HOUSEPLANTS FOR IMPROVING INDOOR AIR QUALITY IN YOUR HOME

✿ALOE (ALOE VERA) EASY-TO-GROW SUCCULENT, GOOD FOR REMOVING FORMALDEHYDE AND BENZENE. ▲

✿SPIDER PLANT (CHLOROPHYTUM COMOSUM) EASY-TO-GROW, GOOD FOR REDUCING BENZENE, FORMALDEHYDE, CARBON MONOXIDE, AND XYLENE.

✿WEEPING FIG (FICUS BENJAMINA) HELPS FILTER OUT FORMALDEHYDE, BENZENE, AND TRICHLOROETHYLENE.

✿CHINESE EVERGREENS (AGLAONEM MODESTUM) LOW-MAINTENANCE PLANT, REMOVES A VARIETY OF AIR POLLUTANTS. ▲

✿RED-EDGED DRACAENA (DRACAENA MARGINATA) SHRUB, GOOD FOR REDUCING XYLENE, TRICHLOROETHYLENE, AND FORMALDEHYDE. ▲

✿HEARTLEAF PHILODENDRON (PHILODENDRON OXYCARDIUM) GREAT FOR REMOVING FORMALDEHYDE AND OTHER TOXINS. ▲ ■

✿RUBBER PLANT (FICUS ELASTICA) A TOUGH PLANT THAT CAN WITHSTAND DIM LIGHT AND COOL TEMPERATURES. GOOD FOR REMOVING FORMALDEHYDE. ▲

✿SNAKE PLANT (SANSEVIERIA TRIFASCIATA 'LAURENTII') ONE OF THE BEST PLANTS FOR REMOVING FORMALDEHYDE. GREAT TO PLACE IN THE BATHROOM. ▲ ■

✿PEACE LILY (SPATHIPHYLLUM) GREAT FOR REMOVING FORMALDEHYDE, BENZENE, AND TRICHLOROETHYLENE. ▲ ■

✿POTHOS (SCINDAPSUS AURES) FAST-GROWING VINE, EFFECTIVE FOR REMOVING FORMALDEHYDE. ▲ ■

✿ENGLISH IVY (HEDERA HELIX) EASY TO GROW AND THRIVES BEST IN MEDIUM TO LOW SUNLIGHT. HELPS REDUCE AIRBORNE FECAL-MATTER PARTICLES. ▲ ■

✿GERBERA DAISY (GERBERA JAMESONII) BEAUTIFUL TO LOOK AT, AND ALSO HELPS REDUCE BENZENE AND TRICHLOROETHYLENE (WHICH CAN COME FROM DRY-CLEANED CLOTHES).

▲ MILD TO SERIOUS TOXICITY TO CATS AND DOGS IF ACCIDENTALLY INGESTED.
■ MILD TO SERIOUS TOXICITY TO SMALL CHILDREN IF ACCIDENTALLY INGESTED.

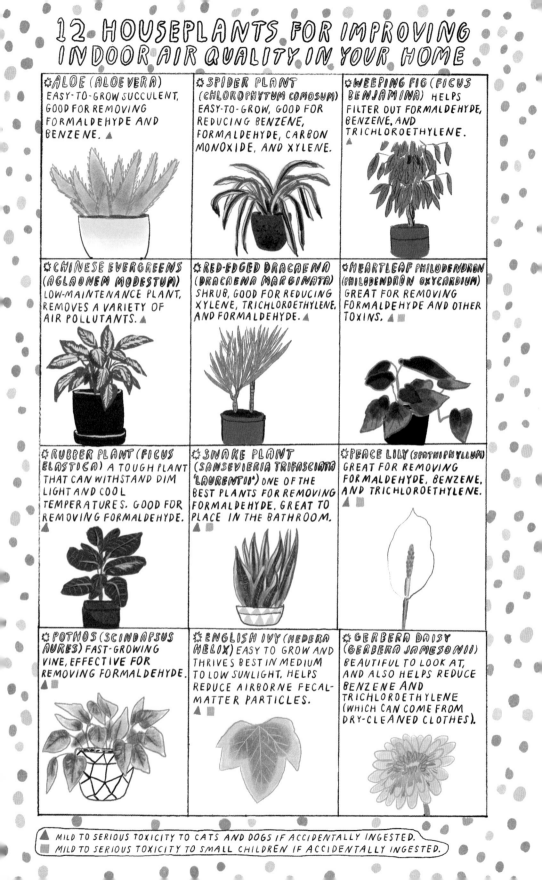

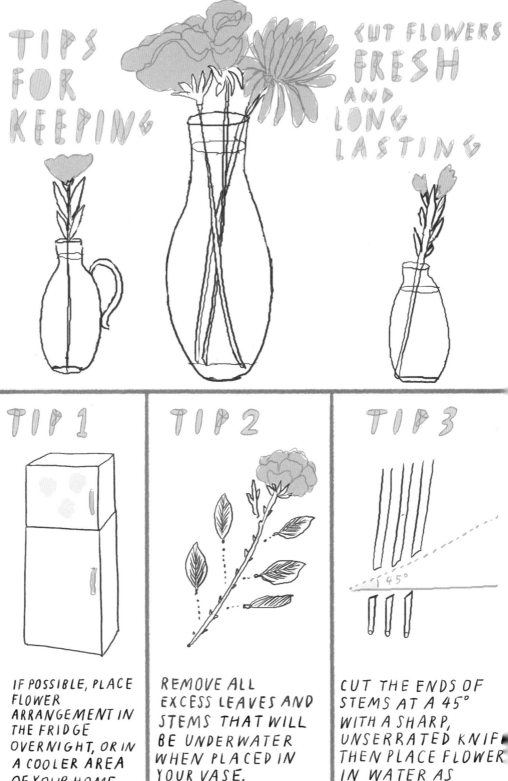

TIPS FOR KEEPING

CUT FLOWERS FRESH AND LONG LASTING

TIP 1

IF POSSIBLE, PLACE FLOWER ARRANGEMENT IN THE FRIDGE OVERNIGHT, OR IN A COOLER AREA OF YOUR HOME.

TIP 2

REMOVE ALL EXCESS LEAVES AND STEMS THAT WILL BE UNDERWATER WHEN PLACED IN YOUR VASE.

TIP 3

45°

CUT THE ENDS OF STEMS AT A 45° WITH A SHARP, UNSERRATED KNIF THEN PLACE FLOWER IN WATER AS QUICKLY AS POSSIBL

TIP 4

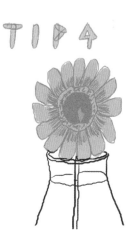

USE COLD WATER, AS PLACING FLOWERS IN LUKEWARM WATER CAN DEHYDRATE THEM.

TIP 5

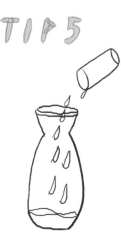

RECUT ENDS OF STEMS EVERY FEW DAYS. CHANGE OUT VASE WATER AT LEAST EVERY OTHER DAY.

TIP 6

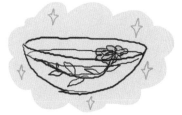

WILTED FLOWERS CAN BE REVIVED BY PLACING THEM IN WARM WATER FOR 30 MINUTES. (THIS TECHNIQUE DOES NOT WORK FOR BULB FLOWERS.)

TIP 7

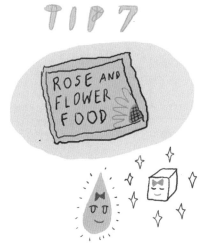

ROSE AND FLOWER FOOD

BE SURE TO ADD FLOWER FOOD TO VASE WATER, AVAILABLE AT FLORIST SHOPS, OR ADD 2 TBS WHITE SUGAR AND 2 TBS APPLE CIDER VINEGAR.

TIP 8

AVOID DIRECT SUNLIGHT, HEAT, AND DRAFTS (SUCH AS FANS), KEEP AWAY FROM FRUIT BOWLS, AS THEY RELEASE ETHYLENE GAS AND CAN EXPEDITE THE WILTING PROCESS.

HOW TO ORGANIZE CHAOTIC CABLE CLUTTER

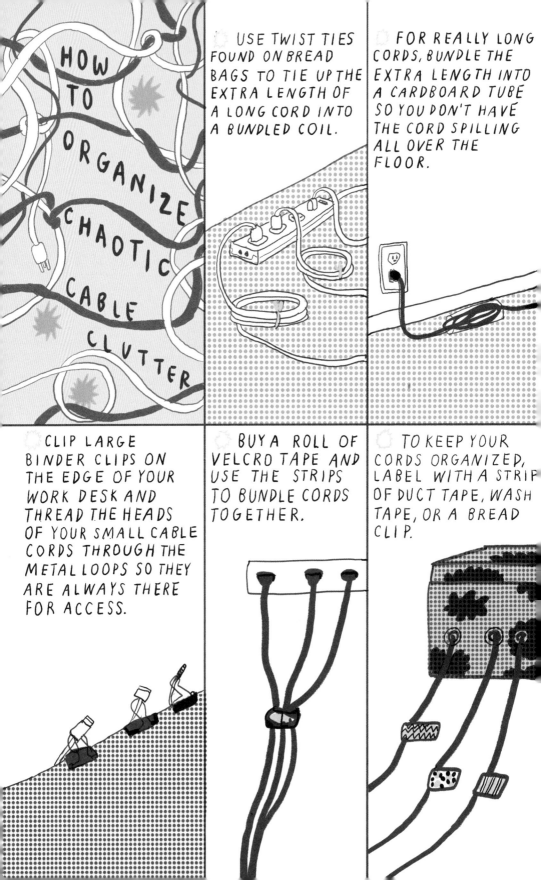

USE TWIST TIES FOUND ON BREAD BAGS TO TIE UP THE EXTRA LENGTH OF A LONG CORD INTO A BUNDLED COIL.

FOR REALLY LONG CORDS, BUNDLE THE EXTRA LENGTH INTO A CARDBOARD TUBE SO YOU DON'T HAVE THE CORD SPILLING ALL OVER THE FLOOR.

CLIP LARGE BINDER CLIPS ON THE EDGE OF YOUR WORK DESK AND THREAD THE HEADS OF YOUR SMALL CABLE CORDS THROUGH THE METAL LOOPS SO THEY ARE ALWAYS THERE FOR ACCESS.

BUY A ROLL OF VELCRO TAPE AND USE THE STRIPS TO BUNDLE CORDS TOGETHER.

TO KEEP YOUR CORDS ORGANIZED, LABEL WITH A STRIP OF DUCT TAPE, WASH TAPE, OR A BREAD CLIP.

KEEP YOUR CORDS BUNDLED TOGETHER BY PUNCHING HOLES THROUGH AN OLD CREDIT CARD AND THREADING CORDS THROUGH HOLES.

HATE THE SIGHT OF YOUR POWER STRIP? PLACE INSIDE A SHOE BOX OR A RIBBON BOX AND CUT HOLES ON THE LONG SIDE WITH A UTILITY KNIFE. THREAD CORDS THROUGH HOLES. DECORATE BOX AS NEEDED.

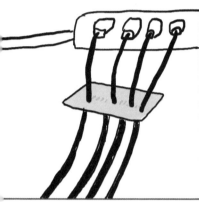

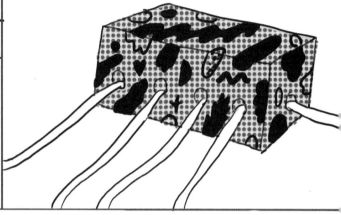

AWESOME STORAGE IDEAS FOR CORDS NOT IN USE:

CD SPINDLES

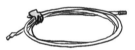

HAIR CLAW (FOR SMALL CORDS)

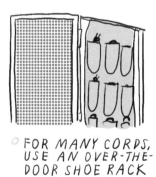

FOR MANY CORDS, USE AN OVER-THE-DOOR SHOE RACK

PLACE CORDS INSIDE PAPER TOWEL ROLLS STORED VERTICALLY IN A BOX

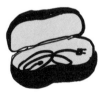

SUNGLASSES CASE (FOR SMALL CORDS ON THE GO)

NIFTY USES FOR WASHI TAPE

WHAT IS WASHI TAPE?

WASHI TAPE IS HIGH-QUALITY DECORATIVE TAPE MADE OF RICE PAPER—IT ORIGINATES FROM JAPAN.

WHY DO PEOPLE LOVE WASHI TAPE?

WASHI TAPE LOOKS PRETTY! ALSO THE ADHESIVE IS NOT TOO STICKY (LIKE THE BACK OF A POST-IT) SO YOU CAN UNSTICK IT, REUSE IT, AND REPOSITION IT ANYTIME.

WHERE TO BUY

WASHI TAPE HAS BECOME SO POPULAR YOU CAN BUY IT AT MOST CRAFT/STATIONERY STORES OR ONLINE.

COOL DECORATION IDEAS

DECORATE THE EXTERIOR OF YOUR IPHONE CASE WITH WASHI TAPE.

LABEL YOUR DIFFERENT CABLE/ COMPUTER CORDS BUT IN A MORE EYE-PLEASING WAY THAN REGULAR LABELS.

COMPUTER KEYBOARD DIRTY OR FADED? COVER WITH WASHI TAPE. (WORKS ESPECIALLY GREAT FOR THE SPACE BAR.)

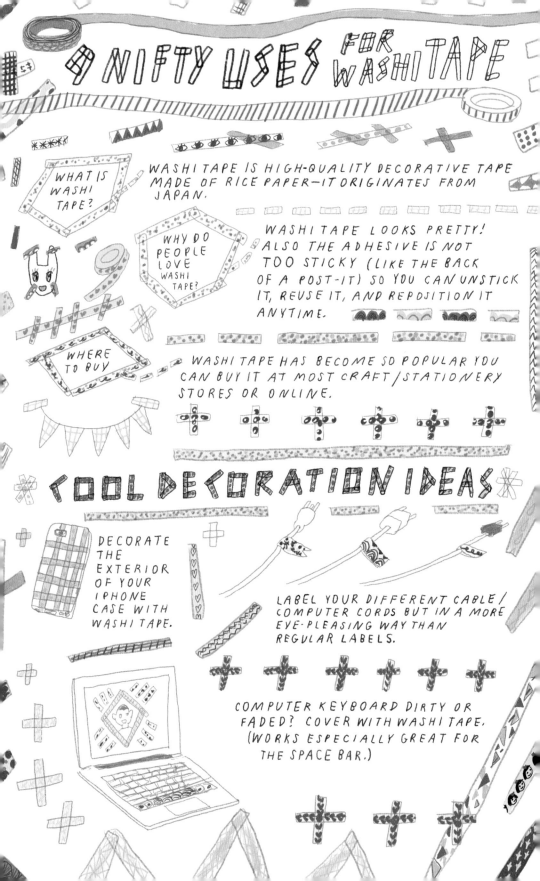

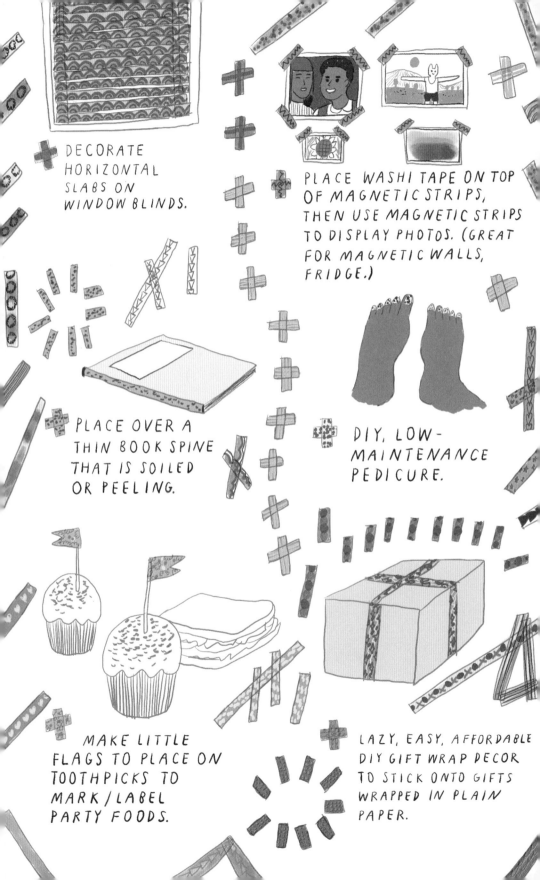

DECORATE HORIZONTAL SLABS ON WINDOW BLINDS.

PLACE WASHI TAPE ON TOP OF MAGNETIC STRIPS, THEN USE MAGNETIC STRIPS TO DISPLAY PHOTOS. (GREAT FOR MAGNETIC WALLS, FRIDGE.)

PLACE OVER A THIN BOOK SPINE THAT IS SOILED OR PEELING.

DIY, LOW-MAINTENANCE PEDICURE.

MAKE LITTLE FLAGS TO PLACE ON TOOTHPICKS TO MARK/LABEL PARTY FOODS.

LAZY, EASY, AFFORDABLE DIY GIFT WRAP DECOR TO STICK ONTO GIFTS WRAPPED IN PLAIN PAPER.

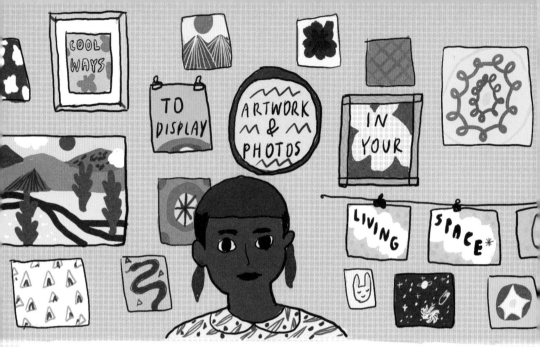

COOL WAYS TO DISPLAY ARTWORK & PHOTOS IN YOUR LIVING SPACE*

* ESPECIALLY IF YOU LIVE IN AN APARTMENT AND YOU DON'T WANT TO MAKE A LOT OF NAIL HOLES IN THE WALLS

✳ PLACE OFFICE BINDER CLIPS ON EACH CORNER OF YOUR PHOTO OR ART PRINT, THEN SECURE TO WALL WITH PUSHPINS OR TACKS.

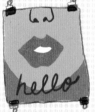

✳ DISPLAY FRAMED PHOTOS/ ARTWORK ON FLOATING SHELVES OR INSIDE BOOKCASES.

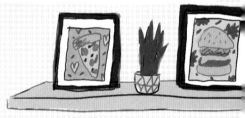

✳ CREATE A FAUX FRAME OUT OF *WASHI TAPE* AND WALL ADHESIVE.

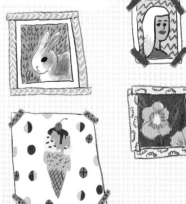

✳ WOODEN PANTS HANGERS ARE A CLEVER WAY TO DISPLAY ART PRINTS.

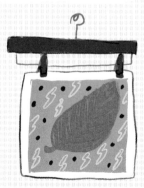

CREATE A "CLOTHESLINE" OF SMALL PHOTOS, POSTCARDS, AND ART PRINTS BY CLIPPING THEM ON A PIECE OF STRING OR TWINE USING SMALL METAL BINDER CLIPS OR CLOTHESPINS. SECURE ENDS OF STRING AGAINST WALL WITH COMMAND HOOKS OR PUSHPINS.

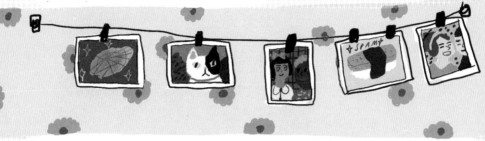

BUY FROM A HARDWARE STORE OR CRAFT STORE A METAL GRID. DEPENDING ON ITS SIZE AND HOW YOU WANT TO USE IT, YOU CAN PROP IT AGAINST A WALL OR HANG IT ABOVE A DESK USING COMMAND HOOKS. USE OFFICE CLIPS TO DISPLAY PHOTOS AND PRINTS.

USING DOUBLE-SIDED ADHESIVE, CREATE A GRID OF POLAROIDS ON A SECTION OF A WALL OR DOOR.

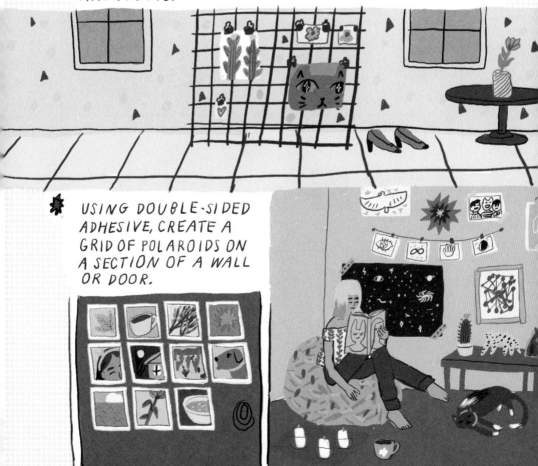

5 FABULOUS IDEAS FOR MAKING YOUR OWN COCKTAIL PARTY-READY DRINK COASTERS

DIY TILE COASTER

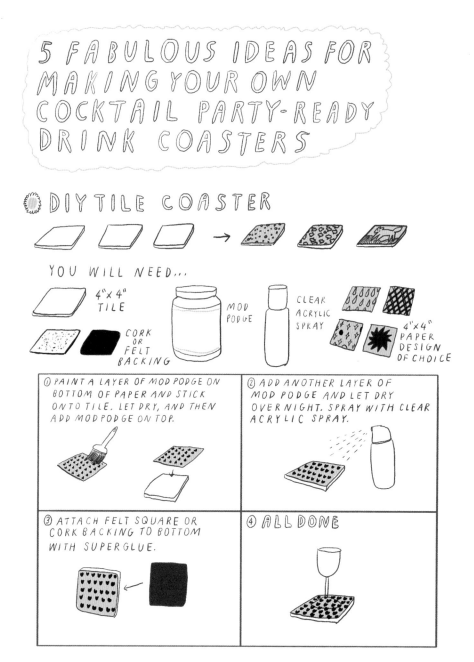

YOU WILL NEED...

4" X 4" TILE

MOD PODGE

CLEAR ACRYLIC SPRAY

CORK OR FELT BACKING

4" X 4" PAPER DESIGN OF CHOICE

① PAINT A LAYER OF MOD PODGE ON BOTTOM OF PAPER AND STICK ONTO TILE. LET DRY, AND THEN ADD MOD PODGE ON TOP.

② ADD ANOTHER LAYER OF MOD PODGE AND LET DRY OVERNIGHT. SPRAY WITH CLEAR ACRYLIC SPRAY.

③ ATTACH FELT SQUARE OR CORK BACKING TO BOTTOM WITH SUPERGLUE.

④ ALL DONE

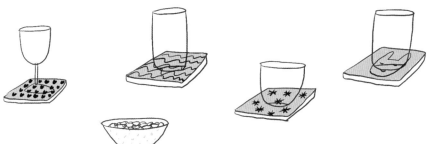

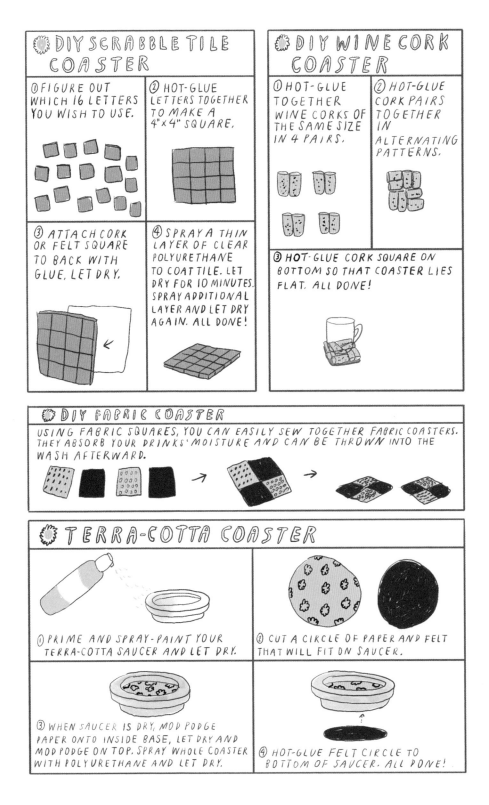

DIY SCRABBLE TILE COASTER

① FIGURE OUT WHICH 16 LETTERS YOU WISH TO USE.

② HOT-GLUE LETTERS TOGETHER TO MAKE A 4"x4" SQUARE.

③ ATTACH CORK OR FELT SQUARE TO BACK WITH GLUE, LET DRY.

④ SPRAY A THIN LAYER OF CLEAR POLYURETHANE TO COAT TILE. LET DRY FOR 10 MINUTES. SPRAY ADDITIONAL LAYER AND LET DRY AGAIN. ALL DONE!

DIY WINE CORK COASTER

① HOT-GLUE TOGETHER WINE CORKS OF THE SAME SIZE IN 4 PAIRS.

② HOT-GLUE CORK PAIRS TOGETHER IN ALTERNATING PATTERNS.

③ HOT-GLUE CORK SQUARE ON BOTTOM SO THAT COASTER LIES FLAT. ALL DONE!

DIY FABRIC COASTER

USING FABRIC SQUARES, YOU CAN EASILY SEW TOGETHER FABRIC COASTERS. THEY ABSORB YOUR DRINKS' MOISTURE AND CAN BE THROWN INTO THE WASH AFTERWARD.

TERRA-COTTA COASTER

① PRIME AND SPRAY-PAINT YOUR TERRA-COTTA SAUCER AND LET DRY.

② CUT A CIRCLE OF PAPER AND FELT THAT WILL FIT ON SAUCER.

③ WHEN SAUCER IS DRY, MOD PODGE PAPER ONTO INSIDE BASE, LET DRY AND MOD PODGE ON TOP. SPRAY WHOLE COASTER WITH POLYURETHANE AND LET DRY.

④ HOT-GLUE FELT CIRCLE TO BOTTOM OF SAUCER. ALL DONE!

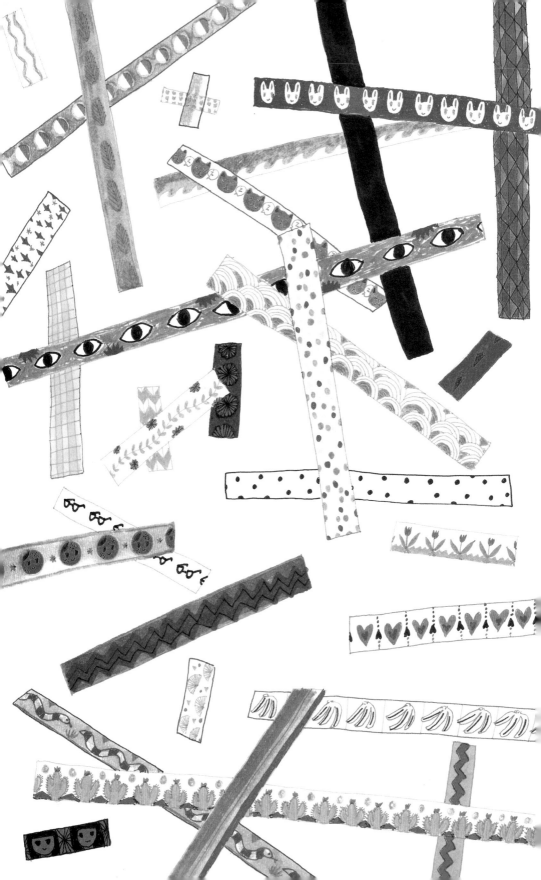

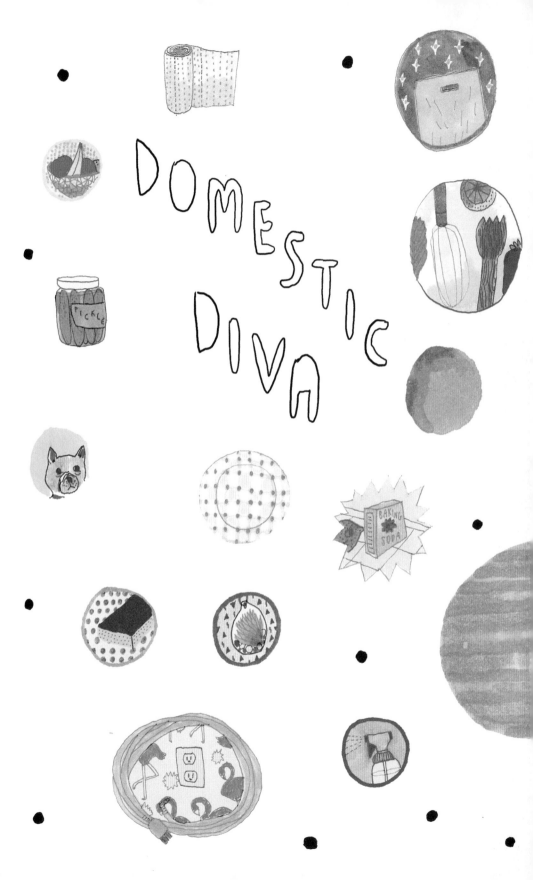

DOMESTIC DIVA

HOW TO ORGANIZE YOUR FRIDGE MORE EFFICIENTLY FOR LONGER-LASTING FOOD

THE IDEAL TEMPERATURE FOR YOUR FRIDGE IS BETWEEN 35°F AND 38°F

NEVER OVERPACK YOUR FRIDGE. THIS OVERWORKS IT AND MAKES IT USE WAY MORE ENERGY.

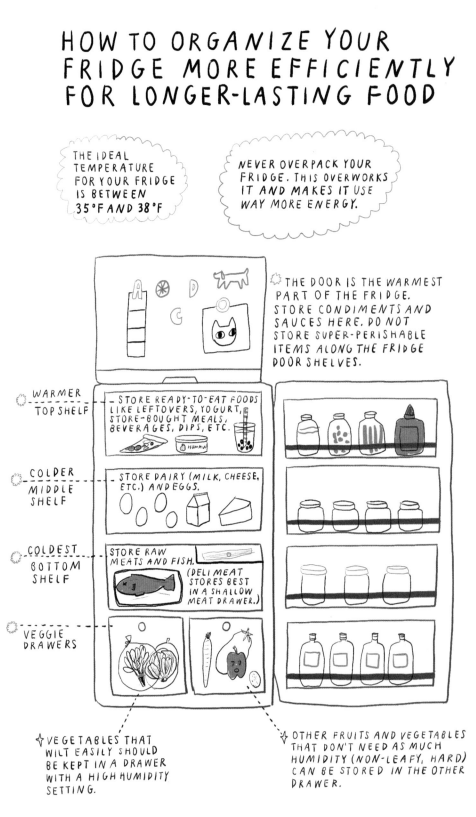

THE DOOR IS THE WARMEST PART OF THE FRIDGE. STORE CONDIMENTS AND SAUCES HERE. DO NOT STORE SUPER-PERISHABLE ITEMS ALONG THE FRIDGE DOOR SHELVES.

WARMER TOP SHELF — STORE READY-TO-EAT FOODS LIKE LEFTOVERS, YOGURT, STORE-BOUGHT MEALS, BEVERAGES, DIPS, ETC.

COLDER MIDDLE SHELF — STORE DAIRY (MILK, CHEESE, ETC.) AND EGGS.

COLDEST BOTTOM SHELF — STORE RAW MEATS AND FISH. (DELI MEAT STORES BEST IN A SHALLOW MEAT DRAWER.)

VEGGIE DRAWERS

VEGETABLES THAT WILT EASILY SHOULD BE KEPT IN A DRAWER WITH A HIGH HUMIDITY SETTING.

OTHER FRUITS AND VEGETABLES THAT DON'T NEED AS MUCH HUMIDITY (NON-LEAFY, HARD) CAN BE STORED IN THE OTHER DRAWER.

1 RUB THE CUT SURFACE OF A LEMON ONTO SURFACE OF CUTTING BOARD WITH A LIBERAL AMOUNT OF SALT. RINSE OFF WITH WATER.

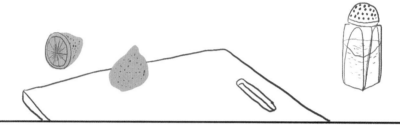

2 SCRUB CUTTING BOARD SURFACE WITH A PASTE MADE FROM 1 TBS BAKING SODA, 1 TBS SALT, AND 1 TBS WATER.

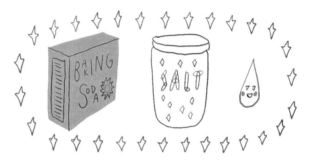

3 SPRAY SURFACE WITH WHITE VINEGAR AND RINSE.

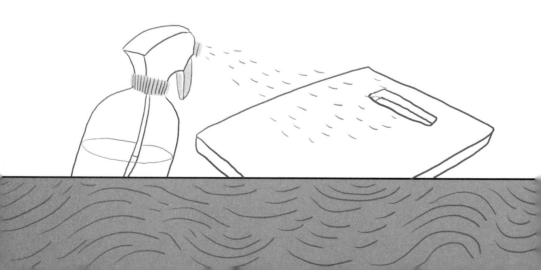

4 WIPE BOARD DOWN WITH A PAPER TOWEL DAMPENED WITH WHITE VINEGAR. RINSE AND WIPE DOWN WITH ANOTHER PAPER TOWEL DAMPENED WITH 3% HYDROGEN PEROXIDE.

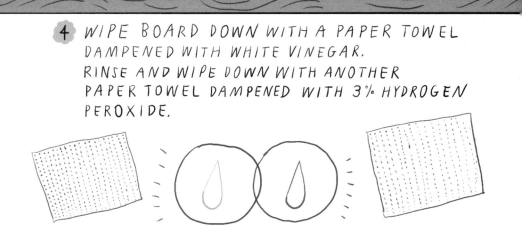

5 SANITIZE CUTTING BOARD USING A SOLUTION OF 1 TSP BLEACH AND 2 QUARTS WATER. FLOOD CUTTING BOARD WITH SOLUTION. LEAVE ON FOR A FEW MINUTES. RINSE THOROUGHLY WITH HOT WATER. THIS IS GREAT FOR CLEANING THE SURFACE AFTER CUTTING RAW MEATS OR SEAFOOD.

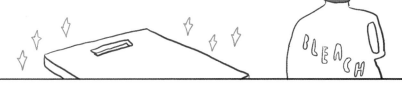

6 DRY BOARD COMPLETELY AND SPRINKLE WITH SALT. SCRUB SURFACE USING A CLEAN SPONGE SOAKED IN HOT WATER AND REPEAT AS NEEDED. GREAT FOR REMOVING STAINS.

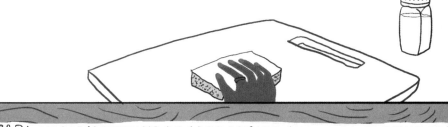

☆TIP☆ WOODEN CUTTING BOARDS SHOULD NEVER BE SUBMERGED IN WATER OR PLACED IN THE DISHWASHER.

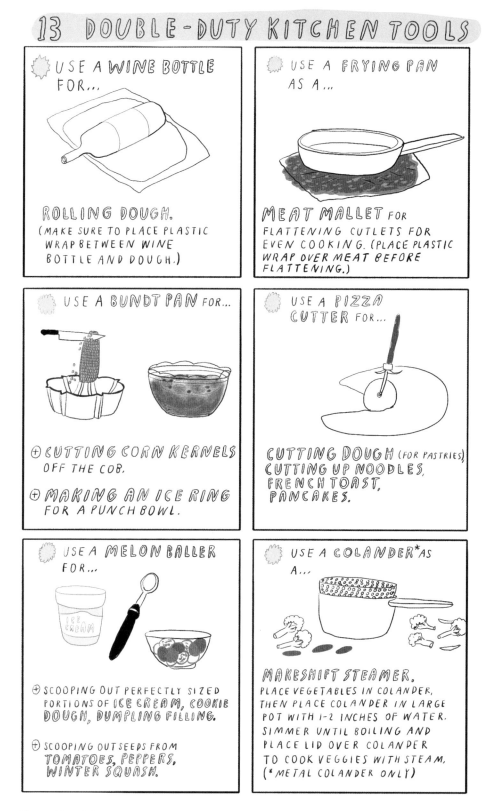

✳ USE A **WINE BOTTLE** FOR...

ROLLING DOUGH.
(MAKE SURE TO PLACE PLASTIC WRAP BETWEEN WINE BOTTLE AND DOUGH.)

✳ USE A **FRYING PAN** AS A...

MEAT MALLET FOR FLATTENING CUTLETS FOR EVEN COOKING. (PLACE PLASTIC WRAP OVER MEAT BEFORE FLATTENING.)

✳ USE A **BUNDT PAN** FOR...

⊕ **CUTTING CORN KERNELS** OFF THE COB.

⊕ **MAKING AN ICE RING** FOR A PUNCH BOWL.

✳ USE A **PIZZA CUTTER** FOR...

CUTTING DOUGH (FOR PASTRIES), **CUTTING UP NOODLES, FRENCH TOAST, PANCAKES.**

✳ USE A **MELON BALLER** FOR...

⊕ SCOOPING OUT PERFECTLY SIZED PORTIONS OF **ICE CREAM, COOKIE DOUGH, DUMPLING FILLING.**

⊕ SCOOPING OUT SEEDS FROM **TOMATOES, PEPPERS, WINTER SQUASH.**

✳ USE A **COLANDER** *AS A...

MAKESHIFT STEAMER.
PLACE VEGETABLES IN COLANDER, THEN PLACE COLANDER IN LARGE POT WITH 1-2 INCHES OF WATER. SIMMER UNTIL BOILING AND PLACE LID OVER COLANDER TO COOK VEGGIES WITH STEAM. (*METAL COLANDER ONLY)

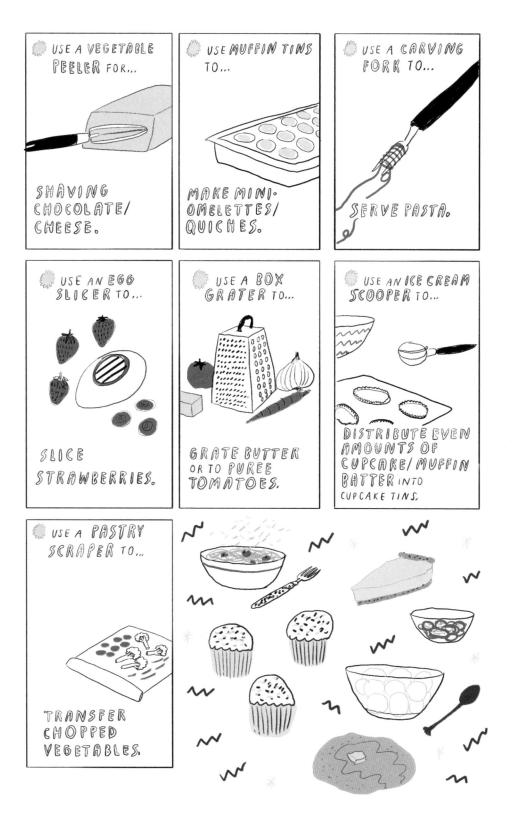

USE A VEGETABLE PEELER FOR...

SHAVING CHOCOLATE/ CHEESE.

USE MUFFIN TINS TO...

MAKE MINI-OMELETTES/ QUICHES.

USE A CARVING FORK TO...

SERVE PASTA.

USE AN EGG SLICER TO...

SLICE STRAWBERRIES.

USE A BOX GRATER TO...

GRATE BUTTER OR TO PUREE TOMATOES.

USE AN ICE CREAM SCOOPER TO...

DISTRIBUTE EVEN AMOUNTS OF CUPCAKE/MUFFIN BATTER INTO CUPCAKE TINS.

USE A PASTRY SCRAPER TO...

TRANSFER CHOPPED VEGETABLES.

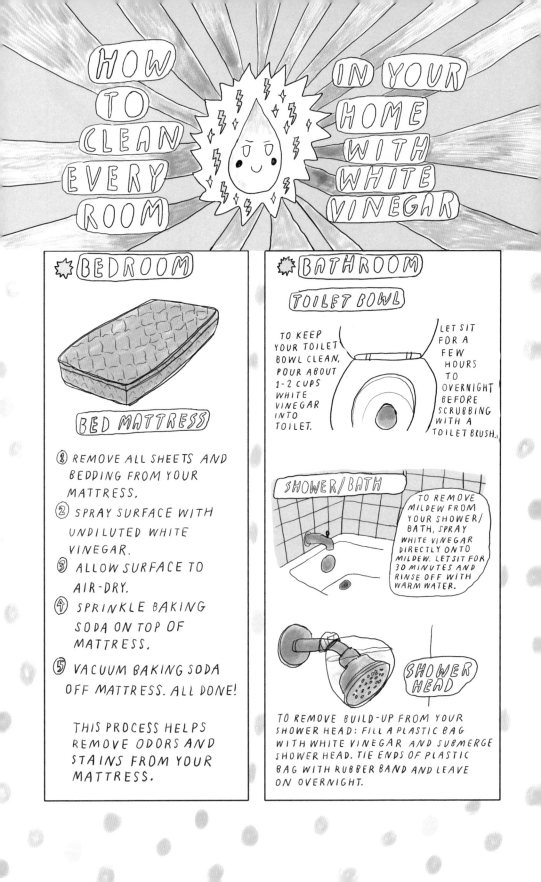

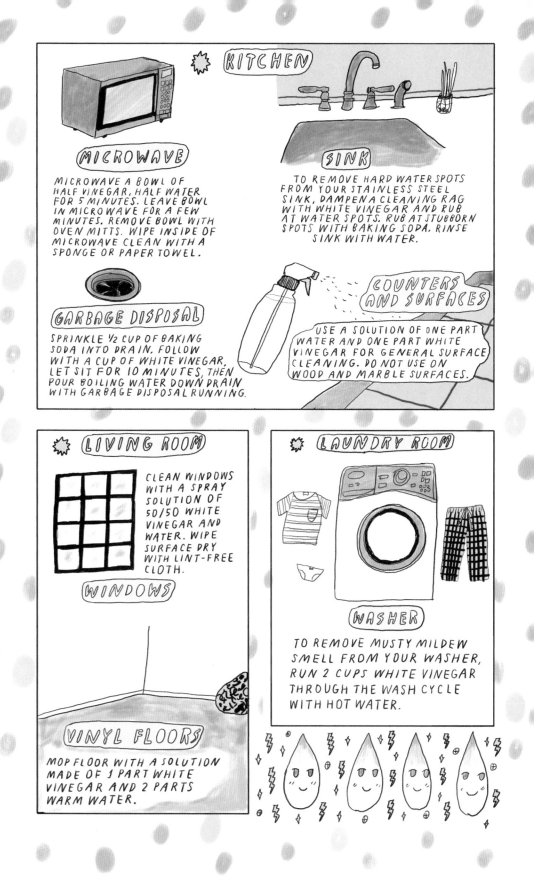

KITCHEN

MICROWAVE

MICROWAVE A BOWL OF HALF VINEGAR, HALF WATER FOR 5 MINUTES. LEAVE BOWL IN MICROWAVE FOR A FEW MINUTES. REMOVE BOWL WITH OVEN MITTS. WIPE INSIDE OF MICROWAVE CLEAN WITH A SPONGE OR PAPER TOWEL.

GARBAGE DISPOSAL

SPRINKLE ½ CUP OF BAKING SODA INTO DRAIN. FOLLOW WITH A CUP OF WHITE VINEGAR, LET SIT FOR 10 MINUTES, THEN POUR BOILING WATER DOWN DRAIN WITH GARBAGE DISPOSAL RUNNING.

SINK

TO REMOVE HARD WATER SPOTS FROM YOUR STAINLESS STEEL SINK, DAMPEN A CLEANING RAG WITH WHITE VINEGAR AND RUB AT WATER SPOTS. RUB AT STUBBORN SPOTS WITH BAKING SODA. RINSE SINK WITH WATER.

COUNTERS AND SURFACES

USE A SOLUTION OF ONE PART WATER AND ONE PART WHITE VINEGAR FOR GENERAL SURFACE CLEANING. DO NOT USE ON WOOD AND MARBLE SURFACES.

LIVING ROOM

CLEAN WINDOWS WITH A SPRAY SOLUTION OF 50/50 WHITE VINEGAR AND WATER. WIPE SURFACE DRY WITH LINT-FREE CLOTH.

WINDOWS

VINYL FLOORS

MOP FLOOR WITH A SOLUTION MADE OF 1 PART WHITE VINEGAR AND 2 PARTS WARM WATER.

LAUNDRY ROOM

WASHER

TO REMOVE MUSTY MILDEW SMELL FROM YOUR WASHER, RUN 2 CUPS WHITE VINEGAR THROUGH THE WASH CYCLE WITH HOT WATER.

HOW TO KEEP YOUR KITCHEN SMELLING FRESH (AND GET RID OF LINGERING BAD/ WEIRD SMELLS)

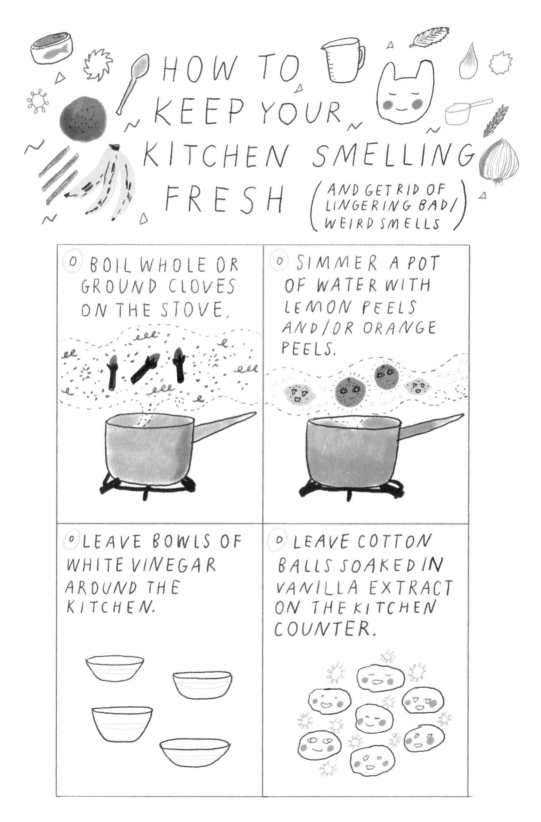

- BOIL WHOLE OR GROUND CLOVES ON THE STOVE.

- SIMMER A POT OF WATER WITH LEMON PEELS AND/OR ORANGE PEELS.

- LEAVE BOWLS OF WHITE VINEGAR AROUND THE KITCHEN.

- LEAVE COTTON BALLS SOAKED IN VANILLA EXTRACT ON THE KITCHEN COUNTER.

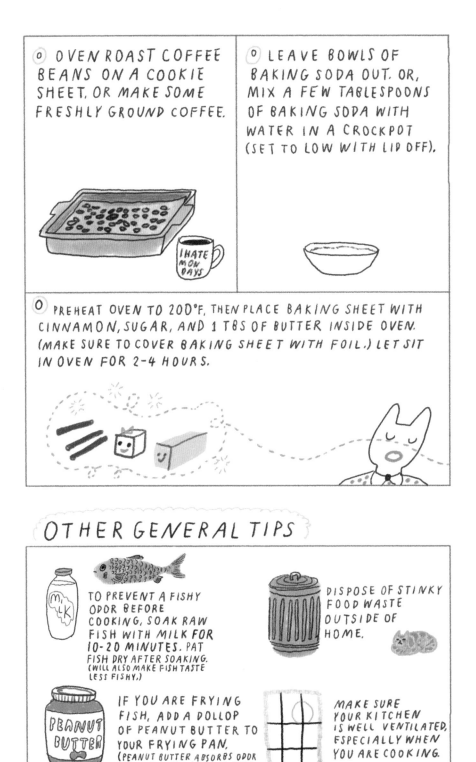

○ OVEN ROAST COFFEE BEANS ON A COOKIE SHEET, OR MAKE SOME FRESHLY GROUND COFFEE.

○ LEAVE BOWLS OF BAKING SODA OUT. OR, MIX A FEW TABLESPOONS OF BAKING SODA WITH WATER IN A CROCKPOT (SET TO LOW WITH LID OFF).

I HATE MONDAYS

○ PREHEAT OVEN TO 200°F, THEN PLACE BAKING SHEET WITH CINNAMON, SUGAR, AND 1 TBS OF BUTTER INSIDE OVEN. (MAKE SURE TO COVER BAKING SHEET WITH FOIL.) LET SIT IN OVEN FOR 2-4 HOURS.

OTHER GENERAL TIPS

TO PREVENT A FISHY ODOR BEFORE COOKING, SOAK RAW FISH WITH MILK FOR 10-20 MINUTES. PAT FISH DRY AFTER SOAKING. (WILL ALSO MAKE FISH TASTE LESS FISHY.)

DISPOSE OF STINKY FOOD WASTE OUTSIDE OF HOME.

IF YOU ARE FRYING FISH, ADD A DOLLOP OF PEANUT BUTTER TO YOUR FRYING PAN. (PEANUT BUTTER ABSORBS ODOR BUT WILL NOT AFFECT FLAVOR OF COOKED FISH.)

MAKE SURE YOUR KITCHEN IS WELL VENTILATED, ESPECIALLY WHEN YOU ARE COOKING.

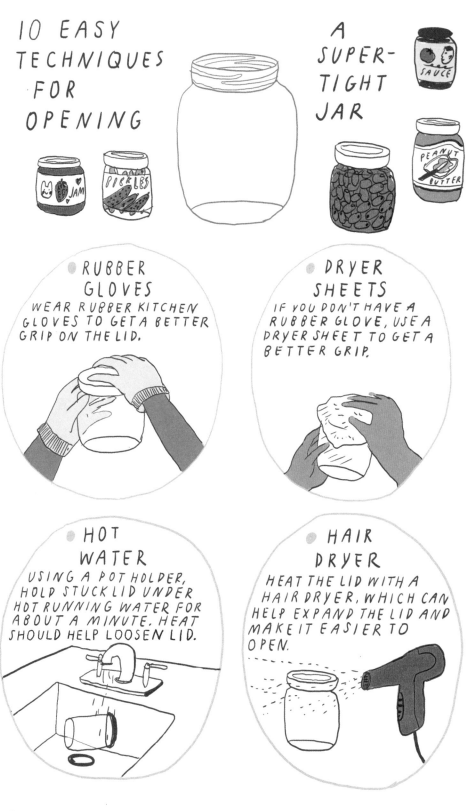

10 EASY TECHNIQUES FOR OPENING

A SUPER-TIGHT JAR

RUBBER GLOVES
WEAR RUBBER KITCHEN GLOVES TO GET A BETTER GRIP ON THE LID.

DRYER SHEETS
IF YOU DON'T HAVE A RUBBER GLOVE, USE A DRYER SHEET TO GET A BETTER GRIP.

HOT WATER
USING A POT HOLDER, HOLD STUCK LID UNDER HOT RUNNING WATER FOR ABOUT A MINUTE. HEAT SHOULD HELP LOOSEN LID.

HAIR DRYER
HEAT THE LID WITH A HAIR DRYER, WHICH CAN HELP EXPAND THE LID AND MAKE IT EASIER TO OPEN.

SCREWDRIVER

SLIDE FLAT HEAD SCREWDRIVER TIP UNDER LID AND USE LEVERAGE TO TRY TO CRACK OPEN SEAL.

RUBBER BANDS

PLACE THICK RUBBER BANDS AROUND LID FOR A BETTER GRIP.

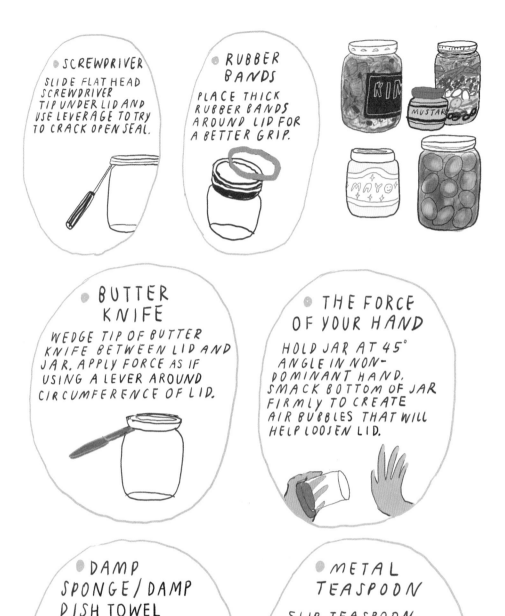

BUTTER KNIFE

WEDGE TIP OF BUTTER KNIFE BETWEEN LID AND JAR. APPLY FORCE AS IF USING A LEVER AROUND CIRCUMFERENCE OF LID.

THE FORCE OF YOUR HAND

HOLD JAR AT 45° ANGLE IN NON-DOMINANT HAND. SMACK BOTTOM OF JAR FIRMLY TO CREATE AIR BUBBLES THAT WILL HELP LOOSEN LID.

DAMP SPONGE/DAMP DISH TOWEL

WRING OUT EXCESS MOISTURE FIRST, THEN USE TO GET A BETTER GRIP ON THE LID.

METAL TEASPOON

SLIP TEASPOON UNDER EDGE OF JAR AND TRY TO BREAK THE SEAL.

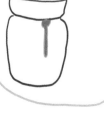

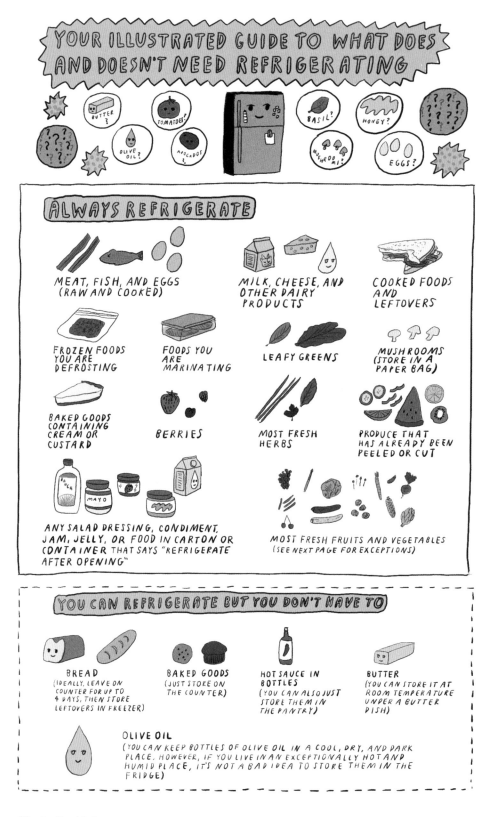

YOUR ILLUSTRATED GUIDE TO WHAT DOES AND DOESN'T NEED REFRIGERATING

BUTTER?
TOMATOES?
OLIVE OIL?
AVOCADOS?
BASIL?
HONEY?
MUSHROOMS?
EGGS?

ALWAYS REFRIGERATE

MEAT, FISH, AND EGGS (RAW AND COOKED)

MILK, CHEESE, AND OTHER DAIRY PRODUCTS

COOKED FOODS AND LEFTOVERS

FROZEN FOODS YOU ARE DEFROSTING

FOODS YOU ARE MARINATING

LEAFY GREENS

MUSHROOMS (STORE IN A PAPER BAG)

BAKED GOODS CONTAINING CREAM OR CUSTARD

BERRIES

MOST FRESH HERBS

PRODUCE THAT HAS ALREADY BEEN PEELED OR CUT

ANY SALAD DRESSING, CONDIMENT, JAM, JELLY, OR FOOD IN CARTON OR CONTAINER THAT SAYS "REFRIGERATE AFTER OPENING"

MOST FRESH FRUITS AND VEGETABLES (SEE NEXT PAGE FOR EXCEPTIONS)

YOU CAN REFRIGERATE BUT YOU DON'T HAVE TO

BREAD (IDEALLY, LEAVE ON COUNTER FOR UP TO 4 DAYS, THEN STORE LEFTOVERS IN FREEZER)

BAKED GOODS (JUST STORE ON THE COUNTER)

HOT SAUCE IN BOTTLES (YOU CAN ALSO JUST STORE THEM IN THE PANTRY)

BUTTER (YOU CAN STORE IT AT ROOM TEMPERATURE UNDER A BUTTER DISH)

OLIVE OIL (YOU CAN KEEP BOTTLES OF OLIVE OIL IN A COOL, DRY, AND DARK PLACE. HOWEVER, IF YOU LIVE IN AN EXCEPTIONALLY HOT AND HUMID PLACE, IT'S NOT A BAD IDEA TO STORE THEM IN THE FRIDGE)

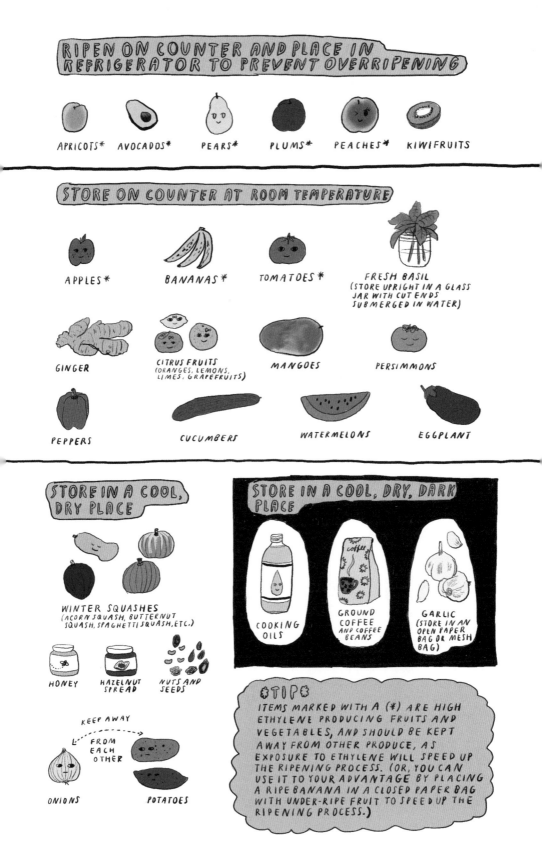

RIPEN ON COUNTER AND PLACE IN REFRIGERATOR TO PREVENT OVERRIPENING

APRICOTS*   AVOCADOS*   PEARS*   PLUMS*   PEACHES*   KIWIFRUITS

STORE ON COUNTER AT ROOM TEMPERATURE

APPLES*   BANANAS*   TOMATOES*   FRESH BASIL
(STORE UPRIGHT IN A GLASS JAR WITH CUT ENDS SUBMERGED IN WATER)

GINGER   CITRUS FRUITS (ORANGES, LEMONS, LIMES, GRAPEFRUITS)   MANGOES   PERSIMMONS

PEPPERS   CUCUMBERS   WATERMELONS   EGGPLANT

STORE IN A COOL, DRY PLACE

WINTER SQUASHES
(ACORN SQUASH, BUTTERNUT SQUASH, SPAGHETTI SQUASH, ETC.)

HONEY   HAZELNUT SPREAD   NUTS AND SEEDS

KEEP AWAY FROM EACH OTHER

ONIONS   POTATOES

STORE IN A COOL, DRY, DARK PLACE

COOKING OILS   GROUND COFFEE AND COFFEE BEANS   GARLIC (STORE IN AN OPEN PAPER BAG OR MESH BAG)

TIP
ITEMS MARKED WITH A (*) ARE HIGH ETHYLENE PRODUCING FRUITS AND VEGETABLES, AND SHOULD BE KEPT AWAY FROM OTHER PRODUCE, AS EXPOSURE TO ETHYLENE WILL SPEED UP THE RIPENING PROCESS. (OR, YOU CAN USE IT TO YOUR ADVANTAGE BY PLACING A RIPE BANANA IN A CLOSED PAPER BAG WITH UNDER-RIPE FRUIT TO SPEED UP THE RIPENING PROCESS.)

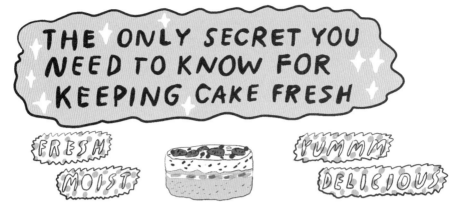

THE ONLY SECRET YOU NEED TO KNOW FOR KEEPING CAKE FRESH

FRESH MOIST

YUMMM DELICIOUS

THE TYPICAL METHOD FOR SLICING A CAKE IS IN TRIANGULAR WEDGES (FOR CIRCULAR CAKES) OR IN A GRID (FOR RECTANGULAR CAKES).

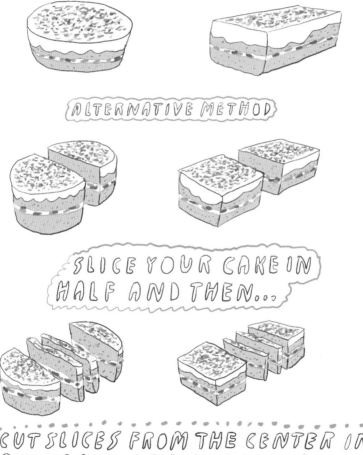

ALTERNATIVE METHOD

SLICE YOUR CAKE IN HALF AND THEN...

CUT SLICES FROM THE CENTER IN RECTANGULAR PORTIONS.

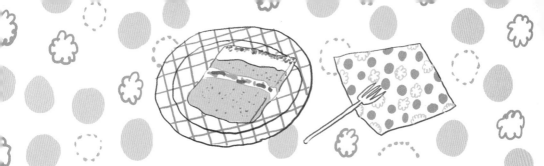

WHEN YOU ARE DONE REMOVING SLICES, SIMPLY TAKE THE TWO LEFTOVER HALVES AND PUSH THEM TOGETHER TO REFORM THE CAKE. THIS WAY, YOU AVOID HAVING DRIED-OUT EDGES.

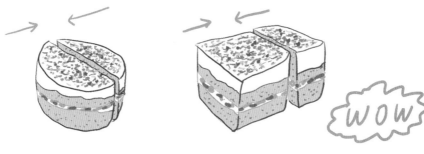

WOW

TIP

FOR EVEN MORE *FRESHNESS* YOU CAN KEEP YOUR CAKE *MOIST* BY ADDING A HALVED APPLE TO YOUR STORAGE CONTAINER. THE MOISTURE FROM THE APPLE WILL PREVENT YOUR CAKE FROM DRYING OUT.

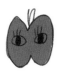

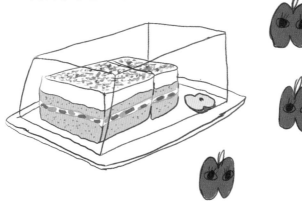

7 REASONS TO BUY SILICONE MUFFIN CUPS

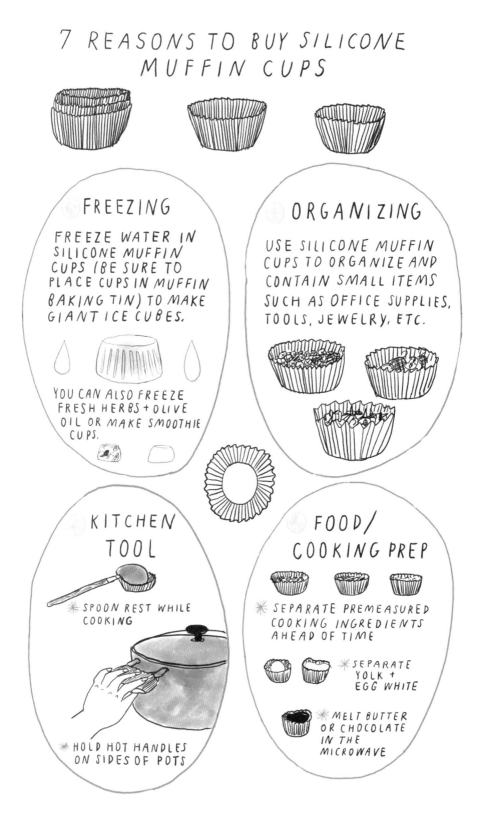

FREEZING

FREEZE WATER IN SILICONE MUFFIN CUPS (BE SURE TO PLACE CUPS IN MUFFIN BAKING TIN) TO MAKE GIANT ICE CUBES.

YOU CAN ALSO FREEZE FRESH HERBS + OLIVE OIL OR MAKE SMOOTHIE CUPS.

ORGANIZING

USE SILICONE MUFFIN CUPS TO ORGANIZE AND CONTAIN SMALL ITEMS SUCH AS OFFICE SUPPLIES, TOOLS, JEWELRY, ETC.

KITCHEN TOOL

✳ SPOON REST WHILE COOKING

✳ HOLD HOT HANDLES ON SIDES OF POTS

FOOD/ COOKING PREP

✳ SEPARATE PREMEASURED COOKING INGREDIENTS AHEAD OF TIME

✳ SEPARATE YOLK + EGG WHITE

✳ MELT BUTTER OR CHOCOLATE IN THE MICROWAVE

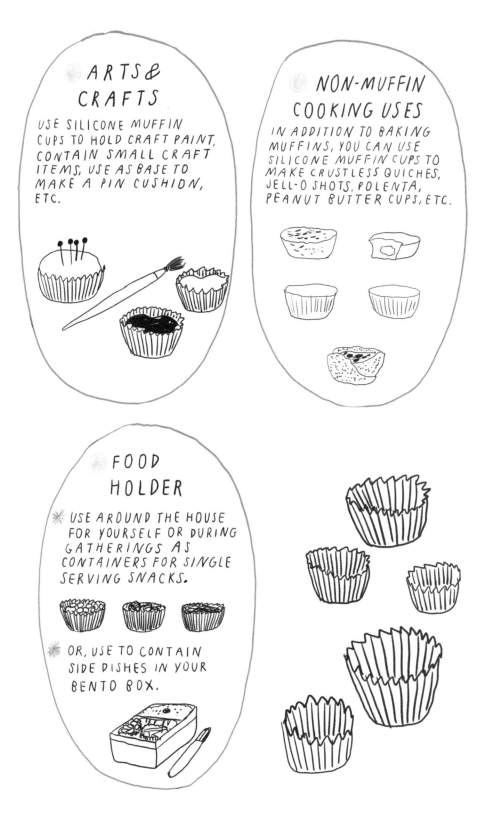

ARTS & CRAFTS

USE SILICONE MUFFIN CUPS TO HOLD CRAFT PAINT, CONTAIN SMALL CRAFT ITEMS, USE AS BASE TO MAKE A PIN CUSHION, ETC.

NON-MUFFIN COOKING USES

IN ADDITION TO BAKING MUFFINS, YOU CAN USE SILICONE MUFFIN CUPS TO MAKE CRUSTLESS QUICHES, JELL-O SHOTS, POLENTA, PEANUT BUTTER CUPS, ETC.

FOOD HOLDER

* USE AROUND THE HOUSE FOR YOURSELF OR DURING GATHERINGS AS CONTAINERS FOR SINGLE SERVING SNACKS.

* OR, USE TO CONTAIN SIDE DISHES IN YOUR BENTO BOX.

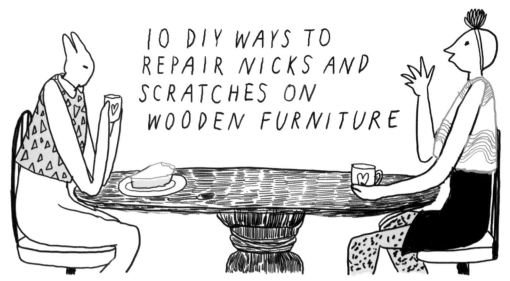

10 DIY WAYS TO REPAIR NICKS AND SCRATCHES ON WOODEN FURNITURE

LEMON JUICE

FOR A MINOR SCRATCH IN THE FINISH, MIX EQUAL PARTS LEMON JUICE AND VEGETABLE OIL. USING A CLEAN LINT-FREE CLOTH, APPLY A GENEROUS AMOUNT AND RUB FIRMLY IN DIRECTION OF SCRATCH UNTIL IT DISAPPEARS.

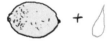

NUTS

USE NUT MEAT TO HIDE THE SCRATCH. RUB THE MEAT OF A BRAZIL NUT / WALNUT / PECAN / ALMOND INTO THE SCRATCH, AND RUB IN THE DIRECTION OF THE SCRATCH.

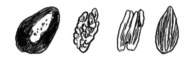

COFFEE GROUNDS

TO DARKEN A LIGHT-COLORED SCRATCH ON WOOD, PLACE COFFEE GROUNDS ON END OF A Q-TIP AND LIGHTLY DAB AT THE SCRATCH. WAIT A FEW HOURS BEFORE APPLYING MORE AS NEEDED.

TEA BAGS

STEEP A BAG OF BLACK TEA IN A FEW TABLESPOONS OF HOT WATER FOR 2-3 MINUTES. DAB TEA INTO SCRATCH WITH A COTTON SWAB AND QUICKLY WIPE AWAY EXCESS WITH A PAPER TOWEL. APPLY MORE AS NEEDED.

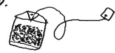

EYEBROW PENCIL

FOR SMALL SCRATCHES, FIND AN EYEBROW PENCIL THAT MATCHES THE COLOR OF THE SURFACE AND FOLLOW THE DIRECTION OF THE SCRATCH.

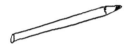

CRAYON

IF YOU HAVE THE RIGHT SHADE OF A WAX CRAYON, USE THAT TO FILL IN THE SCRATCH. WAX CAN EASILY BE REMOVED IF NEEDED.

IODINE

PAINT IODINE IN THE SCRATCH WITH A FINE BRUSH AND ALLOW IT TO DRY. START WITH A LIGHT SHADE BEFORE APPLYING MORE LAYERS. FOR LIGHT-COLORED WOOD, DILUTE IODINE WITH AN EQUAL AMOUNT OF DENATURED ALCOHOL.

ARTIST'S PAINT

USING A COLOR THAT IS DARKER THAN THE FINISH ON THE FURNITURE, APPLY THE OIL-BASED ARTIST'S PAINT INTO THE SCRATCH.

SHOE DYE / SHOE POLISH

YOU CAN USE THE LIQUID FORM OR THE PASTE FORM. USE A FINE BRUSH TO APPLY LIQUID INTO SCRATCH, OR A COTTON SWAB TO APPLY PASTE INTO SCRATCH.

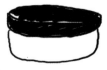

MARKERS

YOU CAN COLOR IN THE SCRATCH WITH A PERMANENT INK FELT-TIP MARKER. FIND THE RIGHT SHADE AT AN ART STORE OR FURNITURE TOUCH-UP MARKERS AT THE HARDWARE STORE.

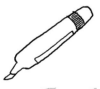

HOW TO MAKE YOUR OWN DIY DISINFECTING WIPES

YOU WILL NEED

STURDY PAPER TOWELS (DON'T GET SUPER-CHEAP BRAND)

MEDIUM-LARGE TUPPERWARE

INGREDIENTS TO CREATE WIPE FLUIDS (SEE NEXT PAGE)

SERRATED KNIFE

SHARP TOOL TO DRILL HOLE

BOWL FOR MIXING

① CUT PAPER TOWEL ROLL TO A SMALLER SIZE THAT WILL FIT YOUR PLASTIC CONTAINER.

② MAKE SURE IT FITS! FOR A CONTAINER, YOU CAN USE A PLASTIC TUPPERWARE OR COFFEE CANISTER.

③ DRILL ½ INCH HOLE IN CENTER OF LID.

④ (ALTERNATELY, YOU CAN MAKE "X" HOLE USING AN X-ACTO KNIFE OR SCISSORS.)

⑤ MAKE YOUR CLEANING SOLUTION. (SEE RECIPES FOR SOME IDEAS.)

⑥ POUR SOLUTION OVER PAPER TOWEL ROLL INSIDE CONTAINER.

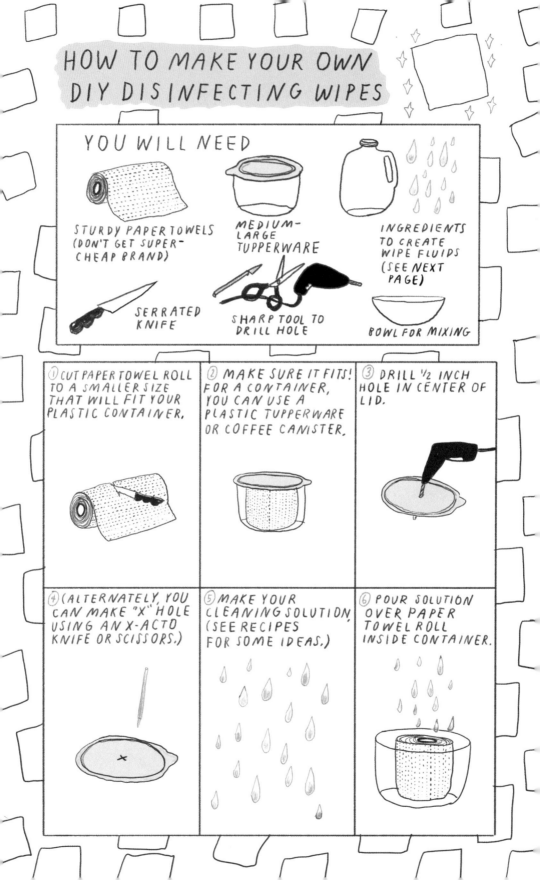

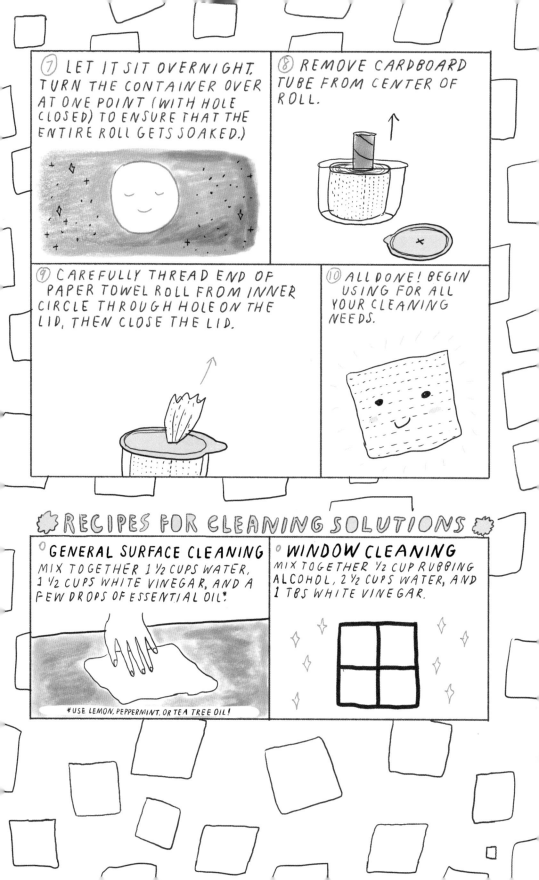

7. LET IT SIT OVERNIGHT. TURN THE CONTAINER OVER AT ONE POINT (WITH HOLE CLOSED) TO ENSURE THAT THE ENTIRE ROLL GETS SOAKED.)

8. REMOVE CARDBOARD TUBE FROM CENTER OF ROLL.

9. CAREFULLY THREAD END OF PAPER TOWEL ROLL FROM INNER CIRCLE THROUGH HOLE ON THE LID, THEN CLOSE THE LID.

10. ALL DONE! BEGIN USING FOR ALL YOUR CLEANING NEEDS.

RECIPES FOR CLEANING SOLUTIONS

GENERAL SURFACE CLEANING
MIX TOGETHER 1½ CUPS WATER, 1½ CUPS WHITE VINEGAR, AND A FEW DROPS OF ESSENTIAL OIL*

*USE LEMON, PEPPERMINT, OR TEA TREE OIL!

WINDOW CLEANING
MIX TOGETHER ½ CUP RUBBING ALCOHOL, 2½ CUPS WATER, AND 1 TBS WHITE VINEGAR.

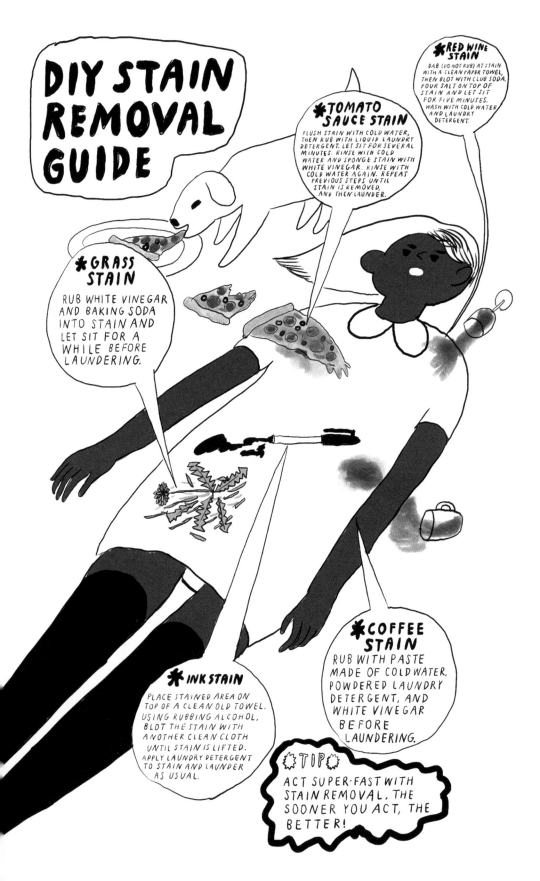

MUD/DIRT STAIN LET MUD STAIN DRY COMPLETELY. REMOVE AS MUCH DRIED MUD FROM SURFACE AS POSSIBLE. SATURATE STAIN IN LIQUID DISH DETERGENT AND SOAK FOR 15 MINUTES. RUB AT STAIN WITH A WET, OLD TOOTHBRUSH ON BOTH SIDES OF FABRIC. REMOVE AS MUCH STAIN AS POSSIBLE BEFORE LAUNDERING.

FOOD OIL/ FOOD GREASE STAIN WIPE UP OIL STAIN AS MUCH AS POSSIBLE WITH A PAPER TOWEL. SATURATE REMAINING STAIN IN BLUE DAWN DISH SOAP, LAUNDER AND HANG-DRY.

CHOCOLATE STAIN LET CHOCOLATE STAIN DRY COMPLETELY AND SCRAPE OFF EXCESS WITH A DULL KNIFE OR SPOON. BLOT WITH DISHWASHING SOAP AND WATER, ADD A FEW DROPS OF AMMONIA FOR MILK CHOCOLATE STAINS, OR A FEW DROPS OF WHITE VINEGAR FOR WHITE CHOCOLATE STAINS. LET SIT FOR 15 MINUTES BEFORE RINSING WITH COLD WATER. LAUNDER AS USUAL.

LIPSTICK STAIN SATURATE WITH HAIRSPRAY AND LET SIT FOR 10 MINUTES. TO REMOVE, DAB WITH DAMP CLOTH AND LAUNDER AS USUAL. FOR EXTRA-STUBBORN STAINS, BLOT STAIN WITH DISHWASHING SOAP AND WATER.

THESE TIPS ARE FOR WASHABLE CLOTHING ONLY. DRY-CLEAN ONLY CLOTHES WITH STAINS SHOULD BE TAKEN TO DRY CLEANERS. NEVER PLACE STAINED CLOTHING IN THE DRYER, AS HEAT WILL COMPLETELY SET THE STAIN.

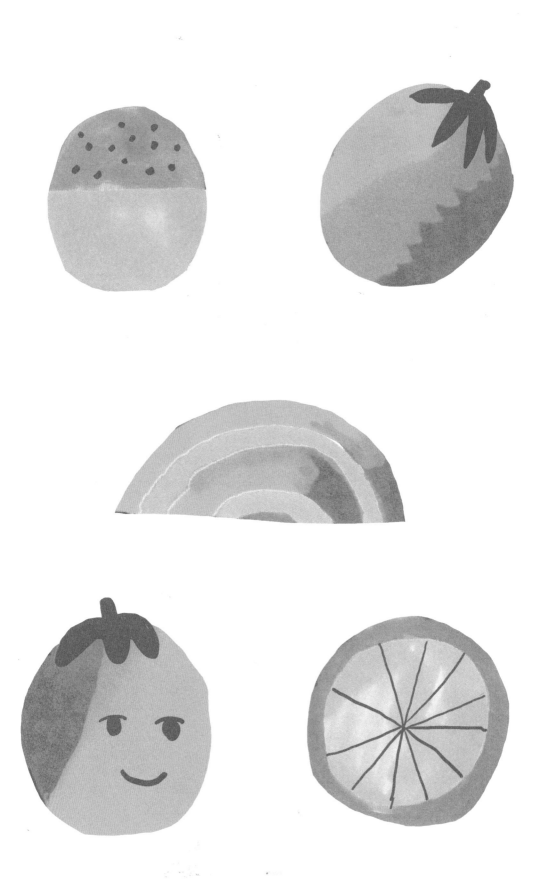

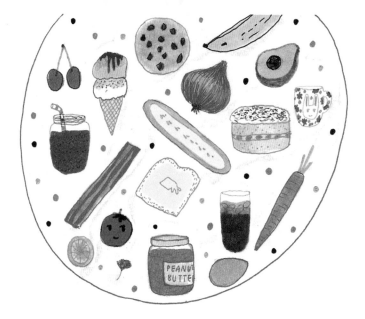

FEED YOURSELF

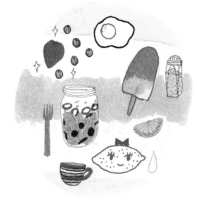

13 HANDY COOKING & BAKING SUBSTITUTIONS FOR MISSING INGREDIENTS

NO SALT?

REPLACE WITH HALF AS MUCH LEMON JUICE. (THIS IS MOSTLY FOR SAVORY COOKING.)

NO GRANULATED SUGAR?

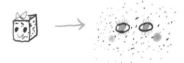

REPLACE 1 CUP GRANULATED SUGAR WITH 1¼ CUP POWDERED SUGAR.

NO CORNSTARCH?

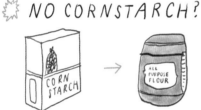

FOR 1 TBS CORNSTARCH, REPLACE WITH 2 TBS ALL-PURPOSE FLOUR OR 1 TBS ARROWROOT POWDER.

NO BREAD CRUMBS?

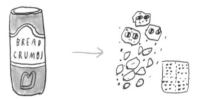

REPLACE WITH SAME AMOUNT OF CRUSHED CRACKER CRUMBS, CORNFLAKES, OR CROUTONS.

NO VANILLA EXTRACT?

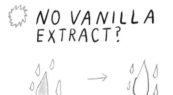

REPLACE WITH HALF AMOUNT OF ALMOND EXTRACT.

NO BUTTER?

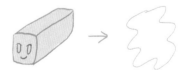

REPLACE 1 CUP WITH 7/8 CUP VEGETABLE OIL OR 1 CUP SHORTENING. ADD ½ TSP SALT FOR REPLACING SALTED BUTTER.

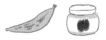 # NO EGG? FOR ONE EGG...

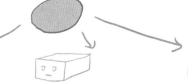

(FOR BAKING SWEETS) REPLACE WITH ½ BANANA OR ¼ CUP UNSWEETENED APPLESAUCE.

(FOR QUICHES & CUSTARDS) REPLACE WITH ¼ CUP SILKEN TOFU AND BLEND WITH OTHER WET INGREDIENTS.

(FOR ALL PURPOSES) REPLACE WITH ¼ CUP EGG SUBSTITUTE.

NO KETCHUP?

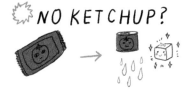

REPLACE 1 CUP KETCHUP WITH 1 CUP TOMATO SAUCE + 1 TSP VINEGAR + 1 TBS SUGAR.

NO SOY SAUCE?

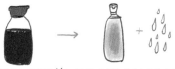

REPLACE ½ CUP SOY SAUCE WITH 4 TBS WORCESTERSHIRE SAUCE MIXED WITH 1 TBS WATER.

NO LEMON?

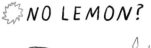
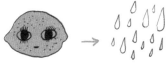

REPLACE 1 TSP LEMON JUICE WITH ½ TSP WHITE VINEGAR.

NO GARLIC?

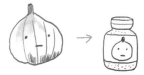

REPLACE 1 CLOVE WITH ½ TSP MINCED GARLIC OR ⅛ TSP GARLIC POWDER.

NO HONEY?

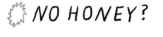
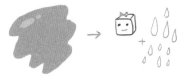

REPLACE 1 CUP HONEY WITH 1¼ CUPS WHITE SUGAR + ⅓ CUP WATER.

NO MAYONNAISE?

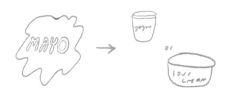

REPLACE 1 CUP MAYONNAISE WITH 1 CUP SOUR CREAM OR 1 CUP PLAIN YOGURT.

12 AWESOME KITCHEN HACKS FOR YOUR NEXT COOKING ADVENTURE

CORE ICEBERG LETTUCE LIKE A BADASS

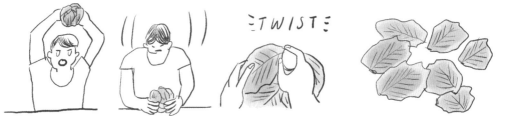

ᴇTWISTᴇ

HOLD THE LETTUCE WITH BOTH HANDS AND SLAM IT, CORE DOWN, AGAINST A HARD AND STURDY SURFACE. GIVE THE CORE A TWIST AND IT SHOULD COME RIGHT OFF.

CUT A BUNCH OF CHERRY TOMATOES AT ONCE

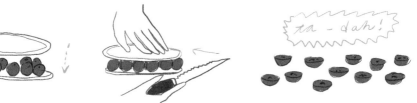

ta - dah!

PLACE CHERRY TOMATOES BETWEEN TWO PLASTIC LIDS. (TAKEOUT CONTAINER LIDS WORK GREAT.) SAW THROUGH GAP WITH A SERRATED KNIFE.

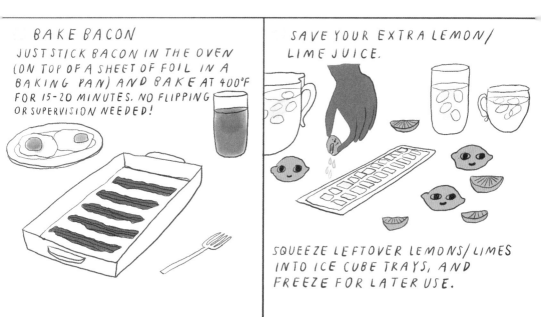

BAKE BACON
JUST STICK BACON IN THE OVEN (ON TOP OF A SHEET OF FOIL IN A BAKING PAN) AND BAKE AT 400°F FOR 15-20 MINUTES. NO FLIPPING OR SUPERVISION NEEDED!

SAVE YOUR EXTRA LEMON/ LIME JUICE.

SQUEEZE LEFTOVER LEMONS/LIMES INTO ICE CUBE TRAYS, AND FREEZE FOR LATER USE.

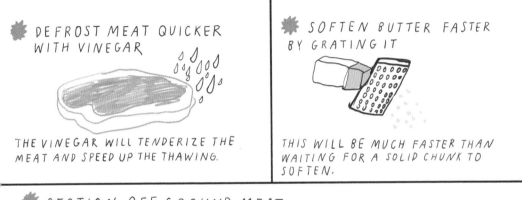

DEFROST MEAT QUICKER WITH VINEGAR

THE VINEGAR WILL TENDERIZE THE MEAT AND SPEED UP THE THAWING.

SOFTEN BUTTER FASTER BY GRATING IT

THIS WILL BE MUCH FASTER THAN WAITING FOR A SOLID CHUNK TO SOFTEN.

SECTION OFF GROUND MEAT

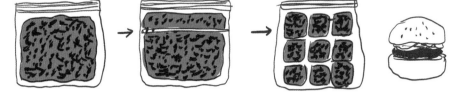

BEFORE PLACING GROUND MEAT IN ZIPLOC BAG IN FREEZER, SECTION IT OFF INTO INDIVIDUAL PORTIONS USING A CHOPSTICK OR RULER.

PREPARE SALAD AHEAD OF TIME WITHOUT MAKING IT SOGGY

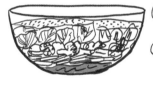

① PLACE SALAD DRESSING AT BOTTOM OF BOWL.

② ON TOP OF THAT, ADD HARD VEGETABLES (CARROTS, BROCCOLI, CELERY, ETC.)

③ ADD THE REST ON TOP. COVER WITH A DAMP PAPER TOWEL. REFRIGERATE FOR UP TO 12 HOURS.

MAKE BREAD RISE FASTER BY SETTING PAN ON TOP OF A HEATING PAD. SIMPLY CRANK HEAT TO HIGH.

WRAP CELERY IN ALUMINUM FOIL TO MAKE IT LAST LONGER. PLACE IN FRIDGE AFTERWARD. CELERY CAN LAST FOR WEEKS.

GRATE GINGER WITH A FORK. MAKE SURE GINGER IS PEELED. NO NEED FOR A GRATER.

CUT ONIONS WITHOUT CRYING

PLACE ONION IN THE FREEZER FOR 15 MINUTES BEFORE CUTTING TO AVOID TEARS.

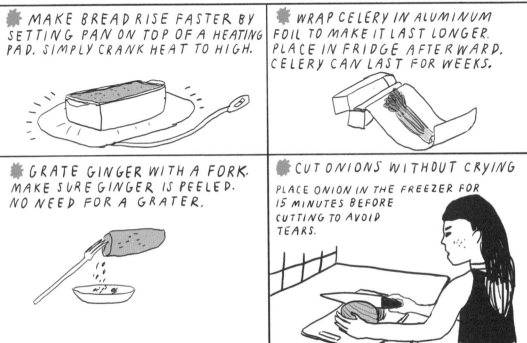

THE BEST WAY TO PEEL A HARD-BOILED EGG

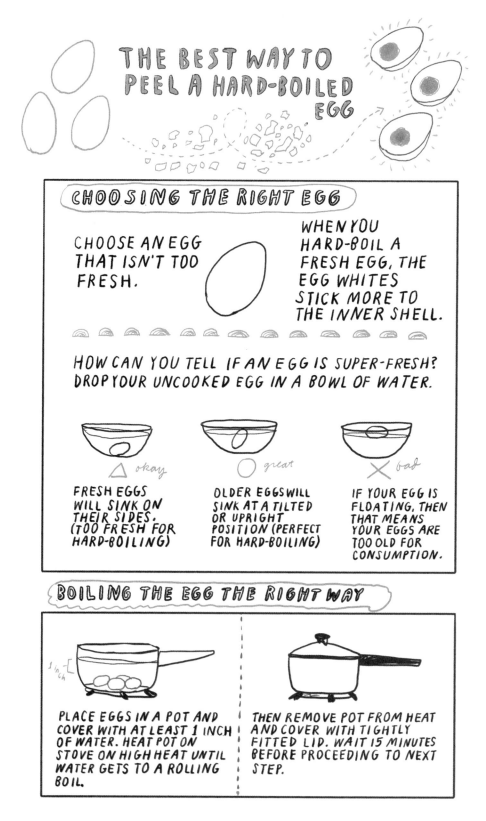

CHOOSING THE RIGHT EGG

CHOOSE AN EGG THAT ISN'T TOO FRESH.

WHEN YOU HARD-BOIL A FRESH EGG, THE EGG WHITES STICK MORE TO THE INNER SHELL.

HOW CAN YOU TELL IF AN EGG IS SUPER-FRESH? DROP YOUR UNCOOKED EGG IN A BOWL OF WATER.

△ okay

FRESH EGGS WILL SINK ON THEIR SIDES. (TOO FRESH FOR HARD-BOILING)

○ great

OLDER EGGS WILL SINK AT A TILTED OR UPRIGHT POSITION (PERFECT FOR HARD-BOILING)

✕ bad

IF YOUR EGG IS FLOATING, THEN THAT MEANS YOUR EGGS ARE TOO OLD FOR CONSUMPTION.

BOILING THE EGG THE RIGHT WAY

PLACE EGGS IN A POT AND COVER WITH AT LEAST 1 INCH OF WATER. HEAT POT ON STOVE ON HIGH HEAT UNTIL WATER GETS TO A ROLLING BOIL.

THEN REMOVE POT FROM HEAT AND COVER WITH TIGHTLY FITTED LID. WAIT 15 MINUTES BEFORE PROCEEDING TO NEXT STEP.

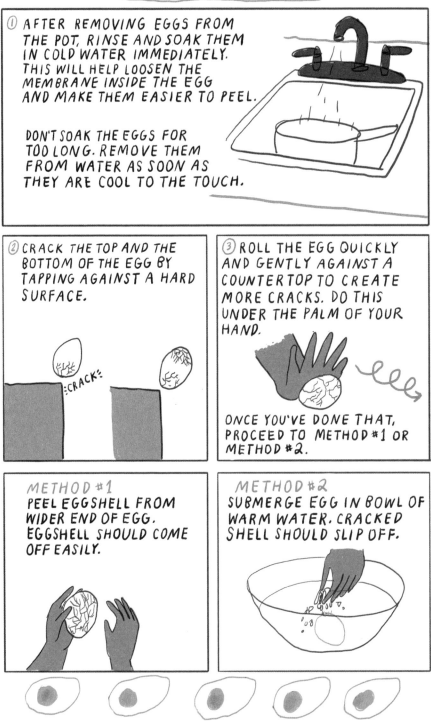

① AFTER REMOVING EGGS FROM THE POT, RINSE AND SOAK THEM IN COLD WATER IMMEDIATELY. THIS WILL HELP LOOSEN THE MEMBRANE INSIDE THE EGG AND MAKE THEM EASIER TO PEEL.

DON'T SOAK THE EGGS FOR TOO LONG. REMOVE THEM FROM WATER AS SOON AS THEY ARE COOL TO THE TOUCH.

② CRACK THE TOP AND THE BOTTOM OF THE EGG BY TAPPING AGAINST A HARD SURFACE.

CRACK!

③ ROLL THE EGG QUICKLY AND GENTLY AGAINST A COUNTERTOP TO CREATE MORE CRACKS. DO THIS UNDER THE PALM OF YOUR HAND.

ONCE YOU'VE DONE THAT, PROCEED TO METHOD #1 OR METHOD #2.

METHOD #1
PEEL EGGSHELL FROM WIDER END OF EGG. EGGSHELL SHOULD COME OFF EASILY.

METHOD #2
SUBMERGE EGG IN BOWL OF WARM WATER. CRACKED SHELL SHOULD SLIP OFF.

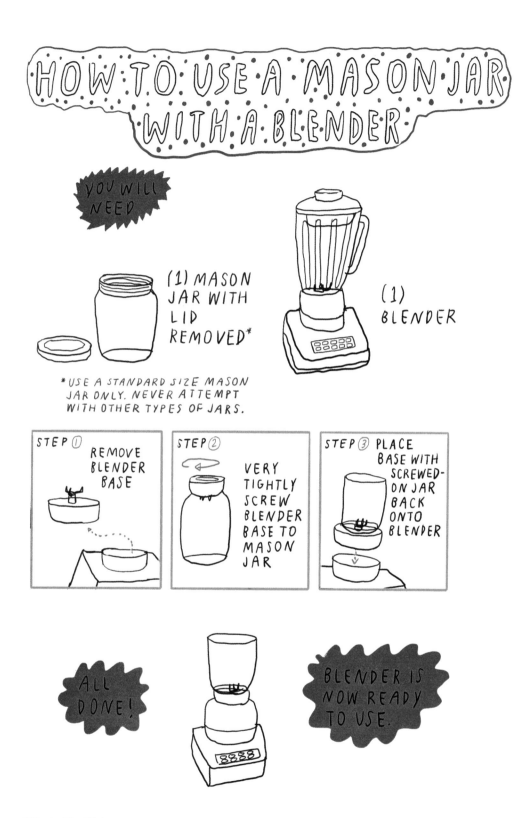

HOW TO USE A MASON JAR WITH A BLENDER

YOU WILL NEED

(1) MASON JAR WITH LID REMOVED*

(1) BLENDER

*USE A STANDARD SIZE MASON JAR ONLY. NEVER ATTEMPT WITH OTHER TYPES OF JARS.

STEP ① REMOVE BLENDER BASE

STEP ② VERY TIGHTLY SCREW BLENDER BASE TO MASON JAR

STEP ③ PLACE BASE WITH SCREWED-ON JAR BACK ONTO BLENDER

ALL DONE!

BLENDER IS NOW READY TO USE.

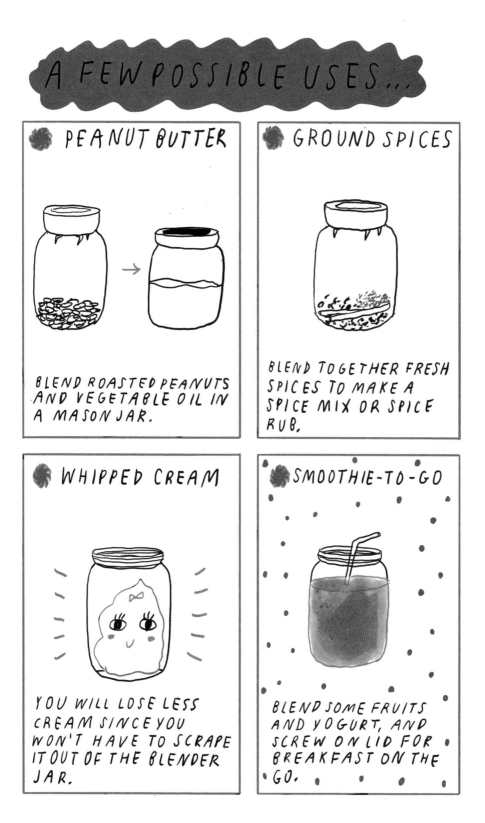

A FEW POSSIBLE USES...

PEANUT BUTTER

BLEND ROASTED PEANUTS AND VEGETABLE OIL IN A MASON JAR.

GROUND SPICES

BLEND TOGETHER FRESH SPICES TO MAKE A SPICE MIX OR SPICE RUB.

WHIPPED CREAM

YOU WILL LOSE LESS CREAM SINCE YOU WON'T HAVE TO SCRAPE IT OUT OF THE BLENDER JAR.

SMOOTHIE-TO-GO

BLEND SOME FRUITS AND YOGURT, AND SCREW ON LID FOR BREAKFAST ON THE GO.

HOW TO MAKE THE PERFECT SCRAMBLED EGGS

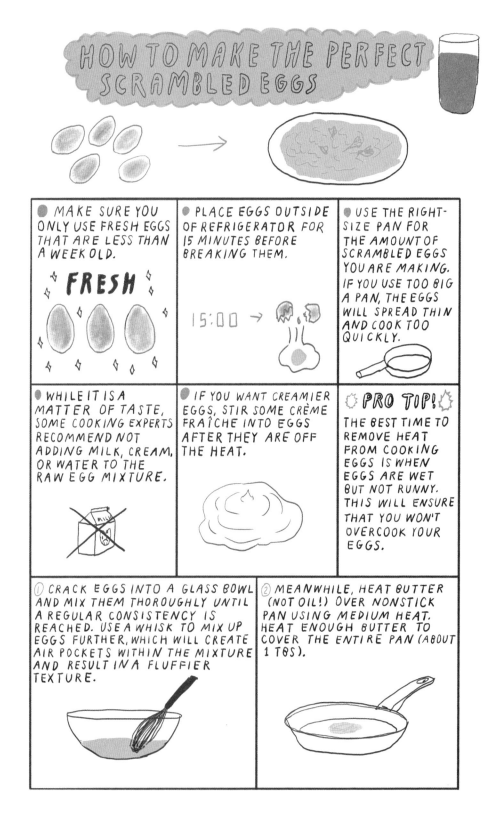

- MAKE SURE YOU ONLY USE FRESH EGGS THAT ARE LESS THAN A WEEK OLD.

FRESH

- PLACE EGGS OUTSIDE OF REFRIGERATOR FOR 15 MINUTES BEFORE BREAKING THEM.

15:00 →

- USE THE RIGHT-SIZE PAN FOR THE AMOUNT OF SCRAMBLED EGGS YOU ARE MAKING. IF YOU USE TOO BIG A PAN, THE EGGS WILL SPREAD THIN AND COOK TOO QUICKLY.

- WHILE IT IS A MATTER OF TASTE, SOME COOKING EXPERTS RECOMMEND NOT ADDING MILK, CREAM, OR WATER TO THE RAW EGG MIXTURE.

- IF YOU WANT CREAMIER EGGS, STIR SOME CRÈME FRAÎCHE INTO EGGS AFTER THEY ARE OFF THE HEAT.

✿ PRO TIP! ✿
THE BEST TIME TO REMOVE HEAT FROM COOKING EGGS IS WHEN EGGS ARE WET BUT NOT RUNNY. THIS WILL ENSURE THAT YOU WON'T OVERCOOK YOUR EGGS.

① CRACK EGGS INTO A GLASS BOWL AND MIX THEM THOROUGHLY UNTIL A REGULAR CONSISTENCY IS REACHED. USE A WHISK TO MIX UP EGGS FURTHER, WHICH WILL CREATE AIR POCKETS WITHIN THE MIXTURE AND RESULT IN A FLUFFIER TEXTURE.

② MEANWHILE, HEAT BUTTER (NOT OIL!) OVER NONSTICK PAN USING MEDIUM HEAT. HEAT ENOUGH BUTTER TO COVER THE ENTIRE PAN (ABOUT 1 TBS).

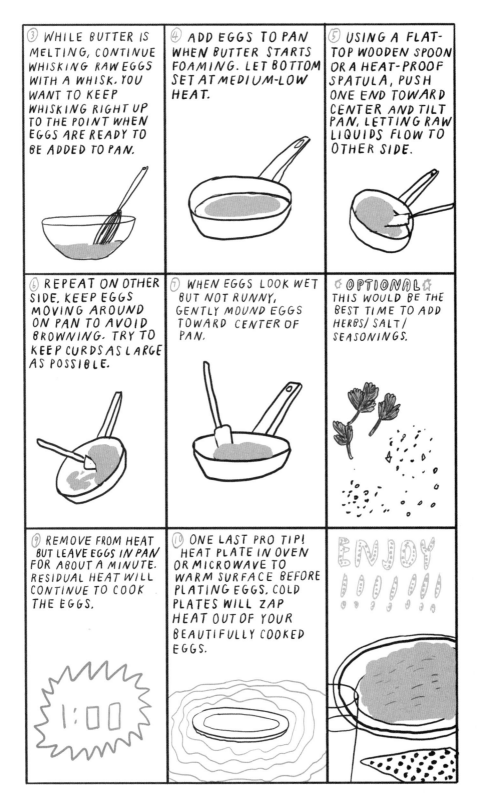

③ WHILE BUTTER IS MELTING, CONTINUE WHISKING RAW EGGS WITH A WHISK. YOU WANT TO KEEP WHISKING RIGHT UP TO THE POINT WHEN EGGS ARE READY TO BE ADDED TO PAN.

④ ADD EGGS TO PAN WHEN BUTTER STARTS FOAMING. LET BOTTOM SET AT MEDIUM-LOW HEAT.

⑤ USING A FLAT-TOP WOODEN SPOON OR A HEAT-PROOF SPATULA, PUSH ONE END TOWARD CENTER AND TILT PAN, LETTING RAW LIQUIDS FLOW TO OTHER SIDE.

⑥ REPEAT ON OTHER SIDE. KEEP EGGS MOVING AROUND ON PAN TO AVOID BROWNING. TRY TO KEEP CURDS AS LARGE AS POSSIBLE.

⑦ WHEN EGGS LOOK WET BUT NOT RUNNY, GENTLY MOUND EGGS TOWARD CENTER OF PAN.

✿ OPTIONAL ✿ THIS WOULD BE THE BEST TIME TO ADD HERBS/SALT/SEASONINGS.

⑨ REMOVE FROM HEAT BUT LEAVE EGGS IN PAN FOR ABOUT A MINUTE. RESIDUAL HEAT WILL CONTINUE TO COOK THE EGGS.

⑩ ONE LAST PRO TIP! HEAT PLATE IN OVEN OR MICROWAVE TO WARM SURFACE BEFORE PLATING EGGS. COLD PLATES WILL ZAP HEAT OUT OF YOUR BEAUTIFULLY COOKED EGGS.

1:00

ENJOY

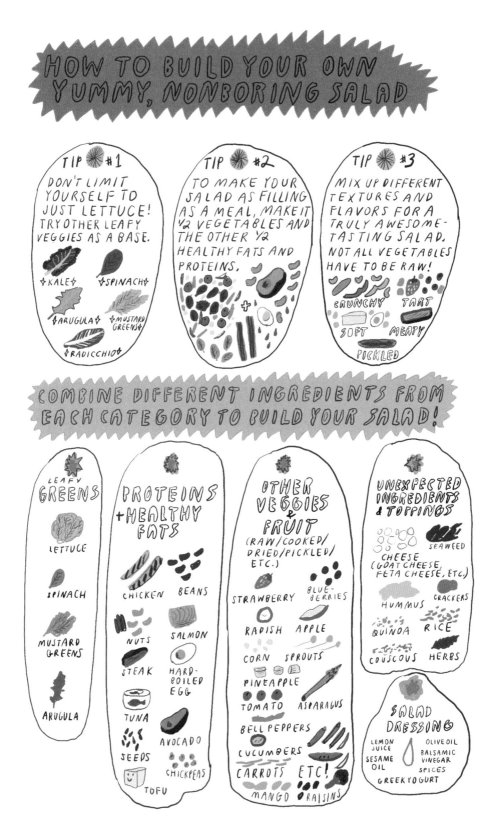

HOW TO BUILD YOUR OWN YUMMY, NONBORING SALAD

TIP #1
DON'T LIMIT YOURSELF TO JUST LETTUCE! TRY OTHER LEAFY VEGGIES AS A BASE.

✧KALE✧ ✧SPINACH✧
✧ARUGULA✧ ✧MUSTARD GREENS✧
✧RADICCHIO✧

TIP #2
TO MAKE YOUR SALAD AS FILLING AS A MEAL, MAKE IT ½ VEGETABLES AND THE OTHER ½ HEALTHY FATS AND PROTEINS.

TIP #3
MIX UP DIFFERENT TEXTURES AND FLAVORS FOR A TRULY AWESOME-TASTING SALAD. NOT ALL VEGETABLES HAVE TO BE RAW!

CRUNCHY TART
SOFT MEATY
PICKLED

COMBINE DIFFERENT INGREDIENTS FROM EACH CATEGORY TO BUILD YOUR SALAD!

LEAFY GREENS
LETTUCE
SPINACH
MUSTARD GREENS
ARUGULA

PROTEINS + HEALTHY FATS
CHICKEN BEANS
NUTS SALMON
STEAK HARD-BOILED EGG
TUNA
SEEDS AVOCADO
CHICKPEAS
TOFU

OTHER VEGGIES & FRUIT
(RAW/COOKED/DRIED/PICKLED/ETC.)
STRAWBERRY BLUEBERRIES
RADISH APPLE
CORN SPROUTS
PINEAPPLE
TOMATO ASPARAGUS
BELL PEPPERS
CUCUMBERS
CARROTS ETC!
MANGO RAISINS

UNEXPECTED INGREDIENTS & TOPPINGS
SEAWEED
CHEESE (GOAT CHEESE, FETA CHEESE, ETC.)
HUMMUS CRACKERS
QUINOA RICE
COUSCOUS HERBS

SALAD DRESSING
LEMON JUICE OLIVE OIL
SESAME OIL BALSAMIC VINEGAR
SPICES
GREEK YOGURT

✳ SOME NONBORING SALAD IDEAS ✳

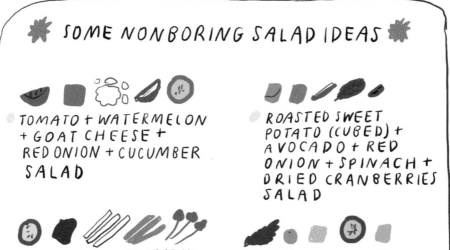

TOMATO + WATERMELON + GOAT CHEESE + RED ONION + CUCUMBER SALAD

ROASTED SWEET POTATO (CUBED) + AVOCADO + RED ONION + SPINACH + DRIED CRANBERRIES SALAD

CUCUMBER + SEAWEED + DAIKON + CARROTS + RADISH SPROUTS SALAD. GREAT WITH SESAME OIL + RICE VINEGAR!

KALE + CHICKPEA + MANGO + CUCUMBER + AVOCADO SALAD. GREAT WITH CITRUSY SALAD DRESSING.

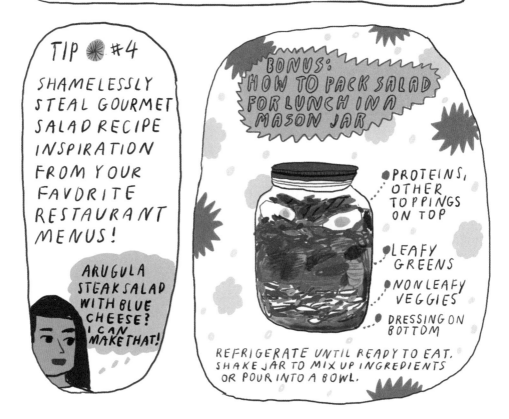

TIP ✳ #4

SHAMELESSLY STEAL GOURMET SALAD RECIPE INSPIRATION FROM YOUR FAVORITE RESTAURANT MENUS!

ARUGULA STEAK SALAD WITH BLUE CHEESE? I CAN MAKE THAT!

BONUS: HOW TO PACK SALAD FOR LUNCH IN A MASON JAR

• PROTEINS, OTHER TOPPINGS ON TOP
• LEAFY GREENS
• NONLEAFY VEGGIES
• DRESSING ON BOTTOM

REFRIGERATE UNTIL READY TO EAT. SHAKE JAR TO MIX UP INGREDIENTS OR POUR INTO A BOWL.

9 SURPRISING USES FOR NUTELLA

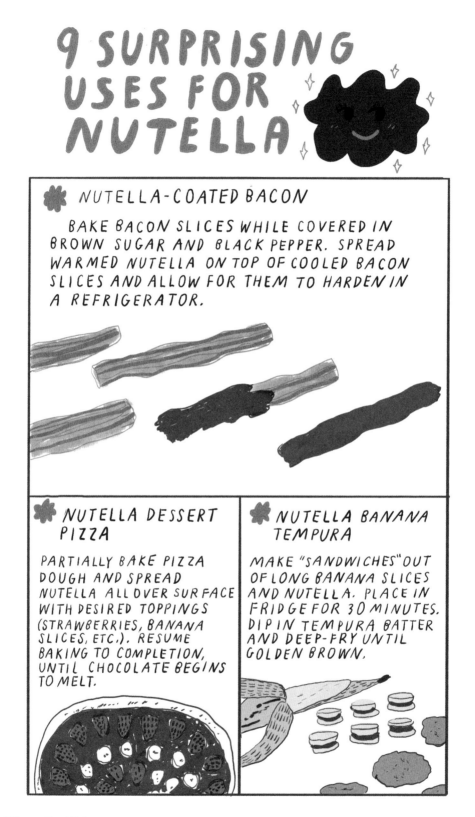

🌸 NUTELLA-COATED BACON

BAKE BACON SLICES WHILE COVERED IN BROWN SUGAR AND BLACK PEPPER. SPREAD WARMED NUTELLA ON TOP OF COOLED BACON SLICES AND ALLOW FOR THEM TO HARDEN IN A REFRIGERATOR.

🌸 NUTELLA DESSERT PIZZA

PARTIALLY BAKE PIZZA DOUGH AND SPREAD NUTELLA ALL OVER SURFACE WITH DESIRED TOPPINGS (STRAWBERRIES, BANANA SLICES, ETC.). RESUME BAKING TO COMPLETION, UNTIL CHOCOLATE BEGINS TO MELT.

🌸 NUTELLA BANANA TEMPURA

MAKE "SANDWICHES" OUT OF LONG BANANA SLICES AND NUTELLA. PLACE IN FRIDGE FOR 30 MINUTES. DIP IN TEMPURA BATTER AND DEEP-FRY UNTIL GOLDEN BROWN.

NUTELLA IN COFFEE

SIMPLY MIX A SPOONFUL INTO YOUR MUG OF COFFEE.

NUTELLA AVOCADO SHAKE

BLEND TOGETHER 1 AVOCADO, 3 TBS CONDENSED MILK, ½ CUP COCONUT MILK, ½ HANDFUL ICE, AND 2 TBS NUTELLA IN A BLENDER.

DIP SALTY POTATO CHIPS IN NUTELLA

NUTELLA AND GRILLED BRIE SANDWICH

SANDWICH NUTELLA AND BRIE BETWEEN TWO SLICES OF BUTTERED CRUSTY FRENCH BREAD. GRILL (TO MAKE THE INSIDES MELTY) AND ENJOY.

SWEET NUTELLA "QUESADILLAS"

MAKE A "QUESADILLA" OUT OF SOFT FLOUR TORTILLAS, NUTELLA, AND YOUR TOPPING OF CHOICE. MICRO-WAVE OR HEAT IN OILED FRYING PAN JUST LONG ENOUGH TO MAKE NUTELLA MELTY.

NUTELLA WONTONS

FILL WONTON WRAPPER WITH 1 TSP NUTELLA AND FOLD INTO A TRIANGLE SHAPE. DEEP-FRY IN VEGETABLE OIL UNTIL GOLDEN BROWN AND DUST WITH POWDERED SUGAR.

THE POSSIBILITIES ARE ENDLESS!

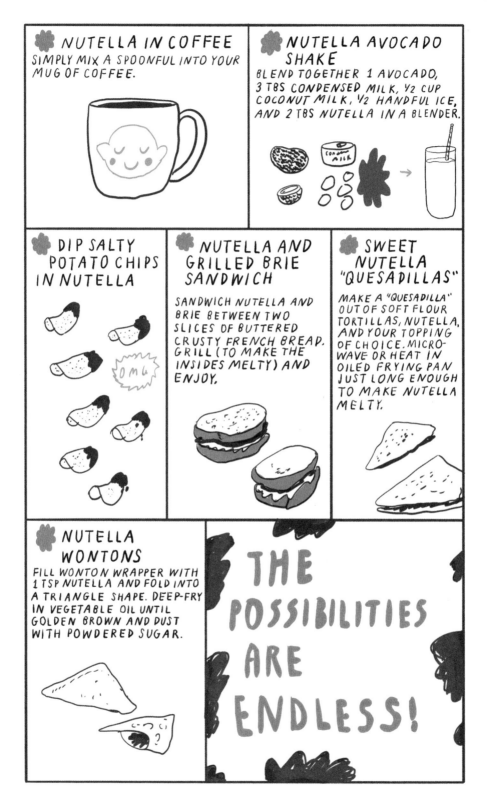

HOW TO MAKE YOUR OWN PEANUT BUTTER

YOU WILL NEED...

2 CUPS PREROASTED, SHELLED PEANUTS (BOTH SALTED AND UNSALTED OKAY).

1 ½ TBS PEANUT OIL

½ TSP SUGAR

PINCH OF KOSHER SALT

① PREHEAT OVEN TO 350°F AND BAKE PEANUTS ON A BAKING PAN FOR 6-8 MINUTES. SHAKE PAN EVERY 2 MINUTES TO AVOID BURNING THEM.

② WAIT FOR THE PEANUTS TO COOL DOWN.

③ POUR PEANUTS INTO A FOOD PROCESSOR WITH METAL BLADES.

④ ADD 1 ½ TBS OIL. (OPTIONAL: ADD 1-2 TBS HONEY FOR A SWEETER FLAVOR.)

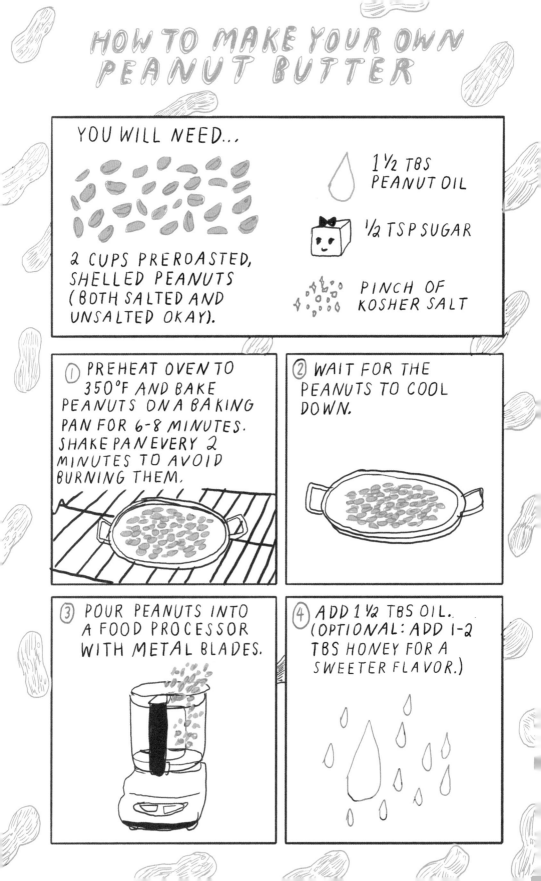

⑤ COVER WITH LID AND CHOP UP PEANUTS FOR 2-3 MINUTES.

3:00

⑥ PERIODICALLY SCRAPE DOWN PEANUTS TOWARD BOTTOM OF FOOD PROCESSOR TO MAKE SURE EVERYTHING GETS CHOPPED UP.

⑦ KEEP PROCESSING UNTIL DESIRED CONSISTENCY IS REACHED. ADD SUGAR AND SALT AS DESIRED FOR OPTIMAL TASTE.

⑧ PLACE IN AIRTIGHT CONTAINER AND REFRIGERATE FOR 1-2 DAYS UNTIL PEANUT BUTTER SETS. ENJOY!

✳ VARIATIONS ✳
FOR A MORE CHOCOLATEY VERSION, ADD ½ CUP UNSWEETENED COCOA POWDER AND 1½ CUPS POWDERED SUGAR WHILE PROCESSING IN THE FOOD PROCESSOR.

ADDITIONALLY, YOU CAN REPLACE THE PEANUT OIL IN THE RECIPE WITH GRAPE-SEED OIL OR COCONUT OIL.

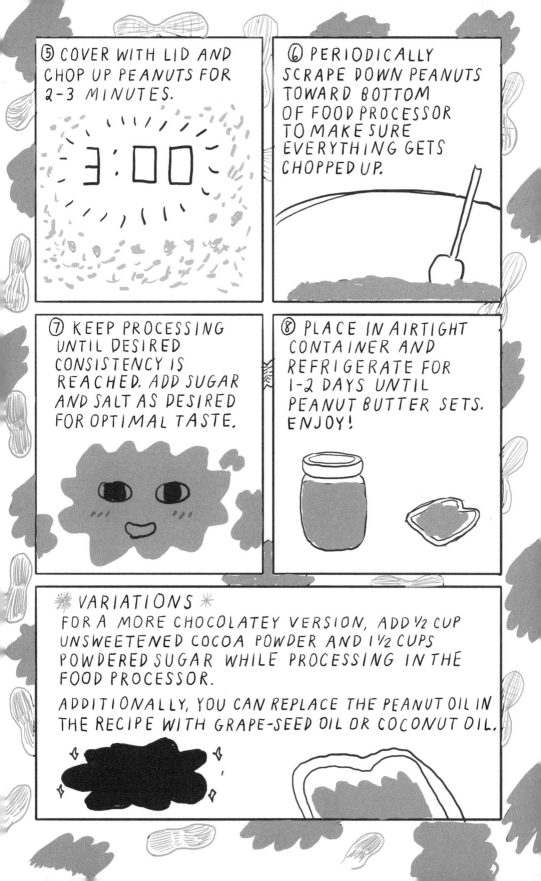

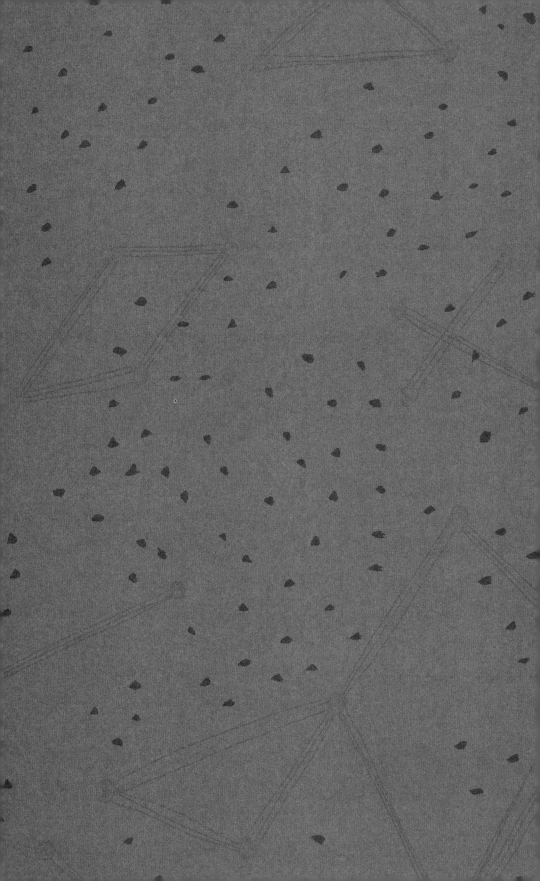

HOW TO MAKE CANDIED BACON

⚙ YOU WILL NEED:

GOOD QUALITY BACON (THICK-CUT WORKS BEST)

BROWN SUGAR

(OPTIONAL) GROUND BLACK PEPPER

① PREHEAT OVEN TO 400 °F.

(oven dial shows 425)

② LINE A SHALLOW BAKING DISH OR BAKING SHEET WITH FOIL. PLACE WIRE COOLING RACK ON TOP.

③ COAT BACON STRIPS WITH BROWN SUGAR BEFORE PLACING THEM SIDE BY SIDE ON COOLING RACK. MAKE SURE THEY DON'T TOUCH EACH OTHER AND THAT BOTH SIDES ARE COATED WELL.

✳ OPTIONAL: ADD BLACK PEPPER TO BROWN SUGAR FOR A MORE PEPPERY KICK.

④ BAKE FOR 20-25 MINUTES IN PREHEATED OVEN, TURNING OVER ONCE. KEEP A CLOSE EYE ON THEM!

20:00

FINISHED CANDIED BACON SHOULD BE CARAMELIZED AND CRISPY-LOOKING, BUT NOT BURNT.

⑤ REMOVE BAKING DISH/SHEET FROM OVEN AND THEN REMOVE BACON FROM COOLING RACK WITH SPATULA WHILE WARM. LET THE CANDIED BACON COOL COMPLETELY AND ENJOY!

SOME DELICIOUS USES FOR CANDIED BACON

⊕ CUPCAKE TOPPING

⊕ IN COOKIES

⊕ IN CHOCOLATE

⊕ ICE CREAM TOPPING (GREAT WITH MAPLE ICE CREAM!)

⊕ ON TOP OF PANCAKES

STORAGE
△ △ △ △ △ △ △

IF YOU ARE USING CANDIED BACON ON THE SAME DAY, COVER WITH PLASTIC WRAP AT ROOM TEMPERATURE UNTIL READY TO USE.

YOU CAN STORE IN THE FRIDGE FOR UP TO A FEW DAYS, BUT TAKE NOTE THAT CANDIED BACON TASTES BEST WHEN EATEN RIGHT AWAY.

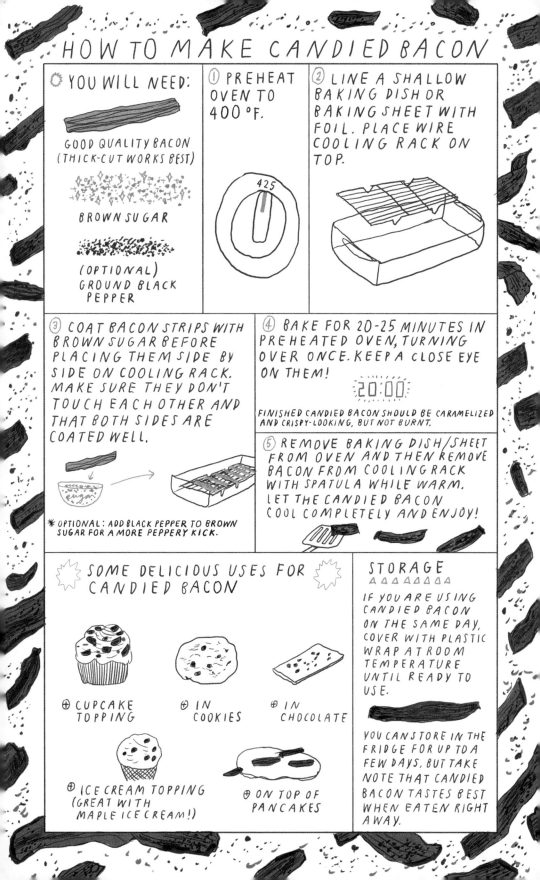

9 EAT ME FLOWERS FOR HAUTE CUISINE

BEGONIAS

YOU CAN SUBSTITUTE THE STEM OF A BEGONIA FOR RHUBARB, OR USE THE FLOWERS AND LEAVES AS GARNISH IN A SALAD.

CHRYSANTHEMUMS

TANGY AND SLIGHTLY BITTER, CHRYSANTHEMUMS ARE BEST LIGHTLY BLANCHED. USE PETALS TO FLAVOR VINEGAR, OR ADD TO SALAD.

DANDELIONS

SWEET AS YOUNG BUDS AND BITTER WHEN MATURE, DANDELIONS CAN BE SERVED RAW OR STEAMED.

DAYLILIES

CAN BE USED AS A COLORFUL GARNISH FOR ANY DISH OR A BEAUTIFUL CAKE TOPPING. HAVE THE SLIGHT SWEETNESS OF ZUCCHINI.

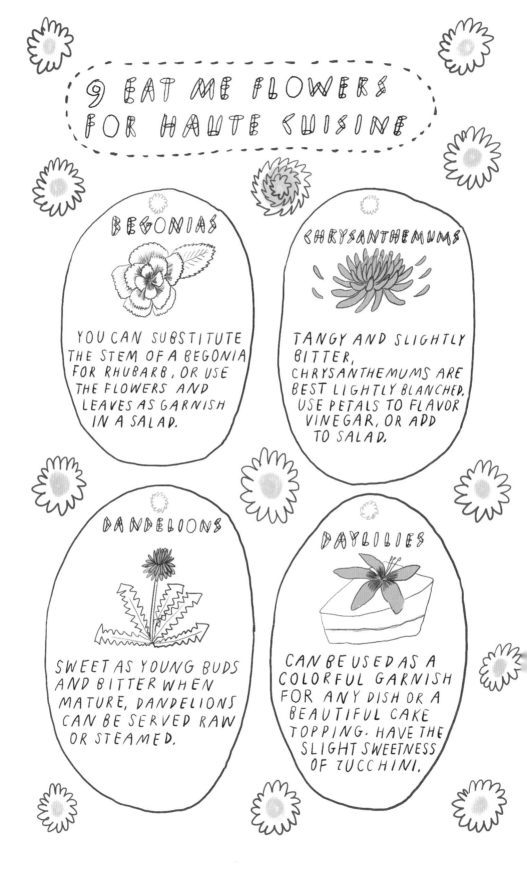

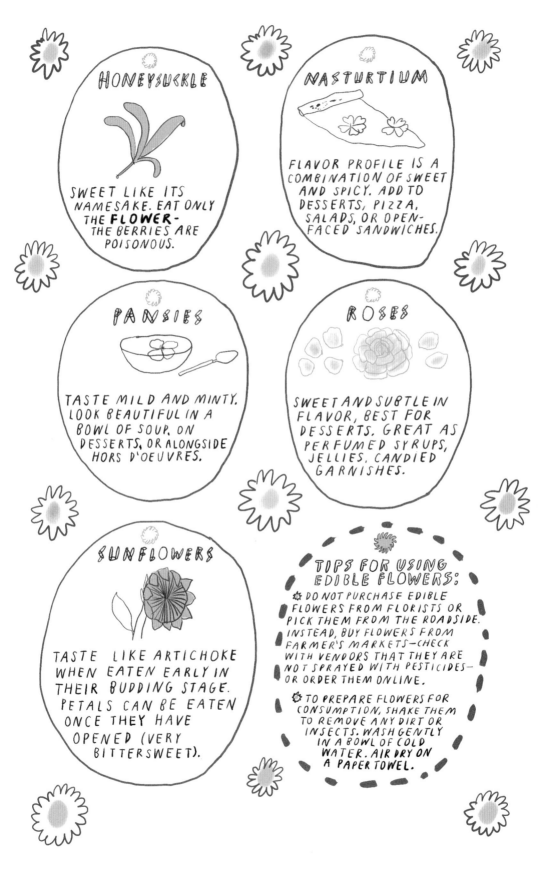

HONEYSUCKLE

SWEET LIKE ITS NAMESAKE. EAT ONLY THE **FLOWER** — THE BERRIES ARE POISONOUS.

NASTURTIUM

FLAVOR PROFILE IS A COMBINATION OF SWEET AND SPICY. ADD TO DESSERTS, PIZZA, SALADS, OR OPEN-FACED SANDWICHES.

PANSIES

TASTE MILD AND MINTY. LOOK BEAUTIFUL IN A BOWL OF SOUP, ON DESSERTS, OR ALONGSIDE HORS D'OEUVRES.

ROSES

SWEET AND SUBTLE IN FLAVOR, BEST FOR DESSERTS. GREAT AS PERFUMED SYRUPS, JELLIES, CANDIED GARNISHES.

SUNFLOWERS

TASTE LIKE ARTICHOKE WHEN EATEN EARLY IN THEIR BUDDING STAGE. PETALS CAN BE EATEN ONCE THEY HAVE OPENED (VERY BITTERSWEET).

TIPS FOR USING EDIBLE FLOWERS:

❀ DO NOT PURCHASE EDIBLE FLOWERS FROM FLORISTS OR PICK THEM FROM THE ROADSIDE. INSTEAD, BUY FLOWERS FROM FARMER'S MARKETS — CHECK WITH VENDORS THAT THEY ARE NOT SPRAYED WITH PESTICIDES — OR ORDER THEM ONLINE.

❀ TO PREPARE FLOWERS FOR CONSUMPTION, SHAKE THEM TO REMOVE ANY DIRT OR INSECTS. WASH GENTLY IN A BOWL OF COLD WATER. AIR DRY ON A PAPER TOWEL.

HOW TO MAKE BROWNIES IN A MUG

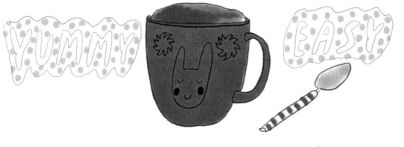

YOU WILL NEED

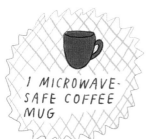

1 MICROWAVE-SAFE COFFEE MUG

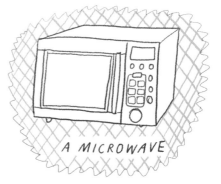

A MICROWAVE

AND THE FOLLOWING INGREDIENTS:

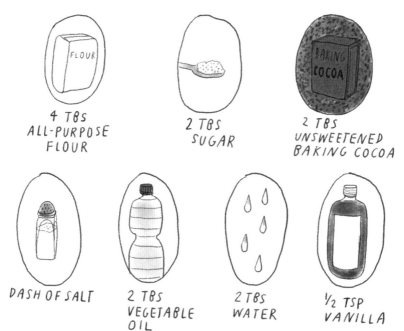

4 TBS ALL-PURPOSE FLOUR

2 TBS SUGAR

2 TBS UNSWEETENED BAKING COCOA

DASH OF SALT

2 TBS VEGETABLE OIL

2 TBS WATER

1/2 TSP VANILLA

① USING A WHISK OR A FORK, MIX TOGETHER THE DRY INGREDIENTS AND THEN ADD THE WET INGREDIENTS UNTIL EVERYTHING IS THOROUGHLY MIXED INTO A MUDLIKE CONSISTENCY.

② (OPTIONAL) FOR A TRULY DECADENT DESSERT, MIX IN A SPOONFUL OF CHOCOLATE CHIPS, PEANUT BUTTER, AND/OR NUTELLA.

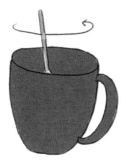

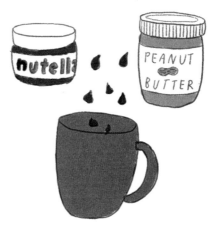

③ MICROWAVE MUG FOR ABOUT 1 MINUTE. DEPENDING ON YOUR MICROWAVE, IDEAL COOKING TIME CAN RANGE FROM 55 SECONDS TO 1 MINUTE 15 SECONDS. CHECK 20-30 SECONDS AT A TIME, FINISHED BROWNIE SHOULD BE A LITTLE WET IN THE CENTER.

④ LET IT COOL FOR ABOUT 1 MINUTE AND DIG IN! BUT DON'T LET IT COOL DOWN FOR TOO LONG OR IT WILL GET SUPER-HARD AND NOT BE AS DELICIOUS. ALSO TASTES DELIGHTFUL WITH A SCOOP OF VANILLA ICE CREAM.

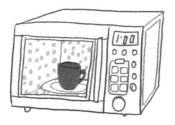

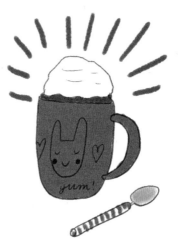

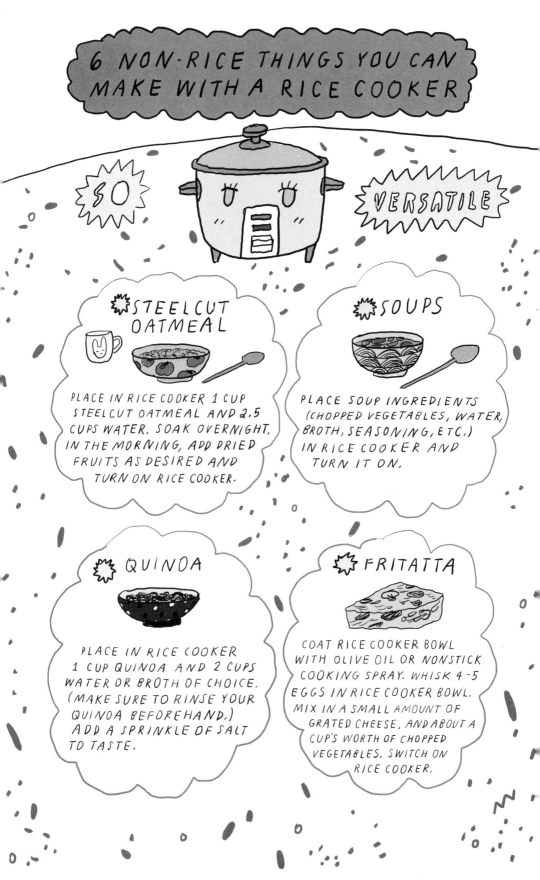

6 NON-RICE THINGS YOU CAN MAKE WITH A RICE COOKER

SO VERSATILE

STEELCUT OATMEAL

PLACE IN RICE COOKER 1 CUP STEELCUT OATMEAL AND 2.5 CUPS WATER. SOAK OVERNIGHT. IN THE MORNING, ADD DRIED FRUITS AS DESIRED AND TURN ON RICE COOKER.

SOUPS

PLACE SOUP INGREDIENTS (CHOPPED VEGETABLES, WATER, BROTH, SEASONING, ETC.) IN RICE COOKER AND TURN IT ON.

QUINOA

PLACE IN RICE COOKER 1 CUP QUINOA AND 2 CUPS WATER OR BROTH OF CHOICE. (MAKE SURE TO RINSE YOUR QUINOA BEFOREHAND.) ADD A SPRINKLE OF SALT TO TASTE.

FRITATTA

COAT RICE COOKER BOWL WITH OLIVE OIL OR NONSTICK COOKING SPRAY. WHISK 4-5 EGGS IN RICE COOKER BOWL. MIX IN A SMALL AMOUNT OF GRATED CHEESE, AND ABOUT A CUP'S WORTH OF CHOPPED VEGETABLES. SWITCH ON RICE COOKER.

STEAMED VEGETABLES

USE A STEAMER RACK OR PLACE UNCOOKED VEGETABLES ON TOP OF RICE IN RICE COOKER TOWARD END OF COOKING CYCLE.

POACHED PEARS

PLACE 3-4 PEELED, HALVED, AND CORED PEARS IN RICE COOKER WITH A FEW CUPS OF JUICE, WINE, OR SUGAR WATER. ADD CINNAMON STICK. COOK FOR ABOUT 30 MINUTES.

MAC AND CHEESE

ADD 2 CUPS ELBOW MACARONI TO 2 CUPS CHICKEN OR VEGETABLE BROTH. CLOSE LID AND COMPLETE ONE RICE COOKER CYCLE, ADD WHOLE MILK (ABOUT 1 CUP), GRATED CHEESE OF CHOICE (ABOUT 1 CUP), KEEP WARM FOR ABOUT 10 MINUTES AND STIR UNTIL DESIRED CREAMINESS / CHEESINESS IS ACHIEVED.

BONUS

YOU CAN USE YOUR RICE COOKER AS A FONDUE POT! USE "KEEP WARM" SETTING TO KEEP FONDUE WARM AND MELTY.

AMAZING!

8 SUPER-EASY AND SUPER-DELICIOUS POPSICLE RECIPES

RECIPES REQUIRE POPSICLE MOLDS

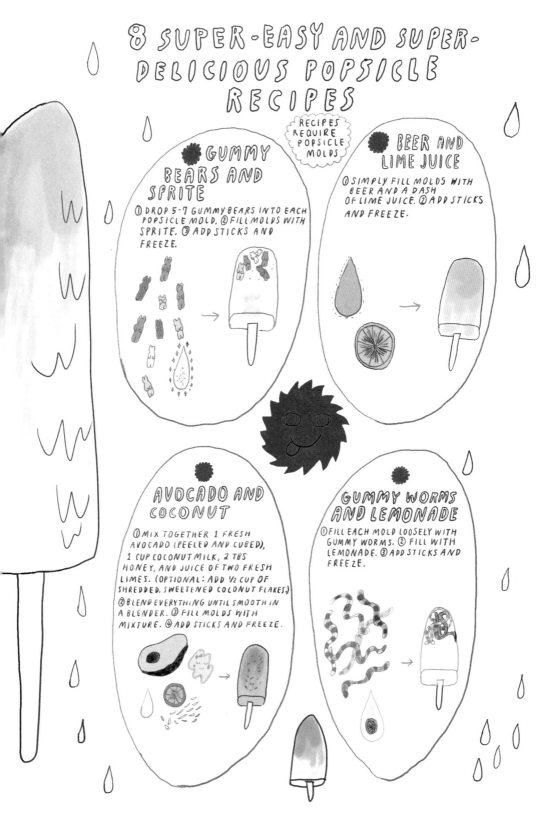

GUMMY BEARS AND SPRITE

① DROP 5-7 GUMMY BEARS INTO EACH POPSICLE MOLD. ② FILL MOLDS WITH SPRITE. ③ ADD STICKS AND FREEZE.

BEER AND LIME JUICE

① SIMPLY FILL MOLDS WITH BEER AND A DASH OF LIME JUICE. ② ADD STICKS AND FREEZE.

AVOCADO AND COCONUT

① MIX TOGETHER 1 FRESH AVOCADO (PEELED AND CUBED), 1 CUP COCONUT MILK, 2 TBS HONEY, AND JUICE OF TWO FRESH LIMES. (OPTIONAL: ADD ½ CUP OF SHREDDED, SWEETENED COCONUT FLAKES.) ② BLEND EVERYTHING UNTIL SMOOTH IN A BLENDER. ③ FILL MOLDS WITH MIXTURE. ④ ADD STICKS AND FREEZE.

GUMMY WORMS AND LEMONADE

① FILL EACH MOLD LOOSELY WITH GUMMY WORMS. ② FILL WITH LEMONADE. ③ ADD STICKS AND FREEZE.

BANANA AND NUTELLA

① BLEND TOGETHER 6 LARGE, OVERRIPE BANANAS UNTIL PUREED. ② ADD ½ CUP NUTELLA AND BLEND UNTIL COMPLETELY MIXED. ③ FILL MOLDS, ADD STICKS, AND FREEZE.

CHOPPED FRUIT AND PUNCH

① PUT SMALL PIECES OF CHOPPED FRUIT IN EACH MOLD. ② FILL WITH FRUIT PUNCH OR 100% WHITE GRAPE JUICE. ③ ADD STICKS AND FREEZE.

TIP: PLACE FROZEN MOLDS UNDER WARM RUNNING WATER FOR ABOUT A MINUTE BEFORE REMOVING POPSICLES.

ICED COFFEE

① MIX TOGETHER 1 CUP COLD BREW COFFEE, 3 TBS SWEETENED CONDENSED MILK, AND 1 CUP MILK. ADD SUGAR AND CREAM TO TASTE. (OPTIONAL: ADD CHOCOLATE CHIPS TO MIXTURE.) ② FILL MOLDS WITH MIXTURE. ③ ADD STICKS AND FREEZE.

OREO POPSICLES

① WHISK TOGETHER 1 3.4OZ PACKAGE VANILLA FLAVOR INSTANT PUDDING, 2 CUPS MILK (WHOLE OR NON-DAIRY), AND ABOUT 8 CRUSHED OREO COOKIES IN A LARGE BOWL. ② FILL MOLDS WITH MIXTURE. ③ ADD STICKS AND FREEZE.

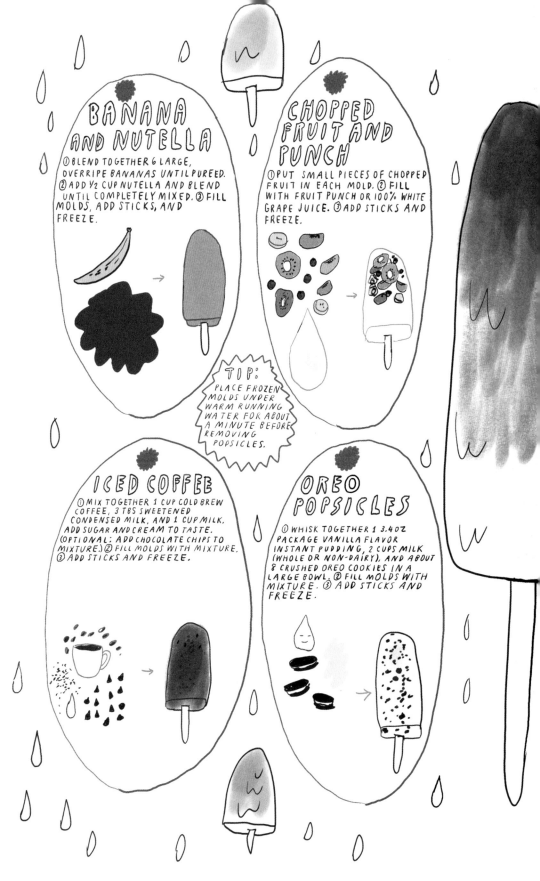

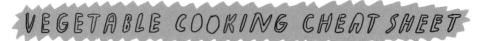

VEGETABLE COOKING CHEAT SHEET

COOKING TIMES CAN VARY DEPENDING ON STOVETOP TEMPERATURE, COOKING EQUIPMENT, ALTITUDE, QUANTITY AND SIZE OF VEGETABLES, ETC. IN GENERAL, COOKED VEGETABLES ARE DONE WHEN THEY ARE TENDER BUT NOT MUSHY. ADJUST ACCORDINGLY TO TASTE.

✳ ARTICHOKES

BOIL: 25-40 MIN
STEAM: 25-40 MIN
SAUTÉ: NOT RECOMMENDED
OVEN ROAST: 425°F, 1 HOUR 15 MIN

✳ ASPARAGUS

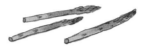

BOIL: 3-5 MIN
STEAM: 6-8 MIN
SAUTÉ: 4-5 MIN
OVEN ROAST: 425°F, 1 HOUR 15 MIN

✳ BEETS

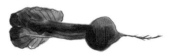

BOIL: 30-60 MIN
STEAM: 40-60 MIN
SAUTÉ: NOT RECOMMENDED
OVEN ROAST: 375°F, 45-60 MIN

✳ BRUSSELS SPROUTS

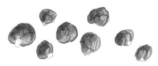

BOIL: 5-10 MIN
STEAM: 6-8 MIN
SAUTÉ: 8-10 MIN
OVEN ROAST: 400°F, 30-40 MIN

✳ BROCCOLI FLORETS

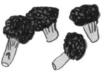

BOIL: 3-5 MIN
STEAM: 4-6 MIN
SAUTÉ: 3-5 MIN
OVEN ROAST: 425°F, 20-25 MIN

✳ CABBAGE
(SHREDDED)

BOIL: 4-7 MIN
STEAM: 3-5 MIN
SAUTÉ: 4-6 MIN
OVEN ROAST: 425°F, 20-30 MIN

✳ CARROTS

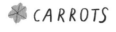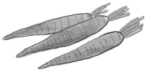

BOIL: 5-10 MIN
STEAM: 4-5 MIN
SAUTÉ: 3-5 MIN
OVEN ROAST: 400°F, 20-25 MIN

✳ CORN ON THE COB
(HUSKS REMOVED)

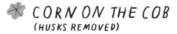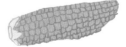

BOIL: 3-5 MIN
STEAM: 4-7 MIN
SAUTÉ: 5-8 MIN
OVEN ROAST: 350°F, 30 MIN

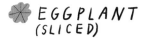 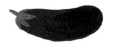 EGGPLANT
(SLICED)

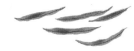 GREEN BEANS

BOIL: 5-10 MIN
STEAM: 10-15 MIN
SAUTÉ: 3-4 MIN
OVEN ROAST: 400°F, 25-30 MIN

BOIL: 10-20 MIN
STEAM: 5-15 MIN
SAUTÉ: 3-4 MIN
OVEN ROAST: 425°F, 12-15 MIN

 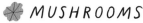 MUSHROOMS

 PEAS

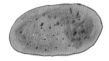

BOIL: 3-4 MIN
STEAM: 5-8 MIN
SAUTÉ: 3-5 MIN
OVEN ROAST: 425°F, 30-35 MIN

BOIL: 2-3 MIN
STEAM: 1-2 MIN
SAUTÉ: 2-3 MIN
OVEN ROAST: NOT
RECOMMENDED ON THEIR OWN,
BUT GREAT WHEN BAKED WITH OTHER
INGREDIENTS (LIKE OVEN-ROASTED POTATOES
AND PEAS, ETC.)!

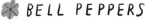 BELL PEPPERS

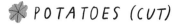 POTATOES (CUT)

BOIL: 4-6 MIN
STEAM: 5-7 MIN
SAUTÉ: 7-10 MIN
OVEN ROAST: 450°F, 50-60 MIN

BOIL: 15-20 MIN
STEAM: 10-20 MIN
SAUTÉ: 10-15 MIN
OVEN ROAST: 400°F, 45-60 MIN

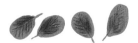 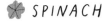 SPINACH

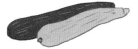 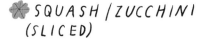 SQUASH / ZUCCHINI
(SLICED)

BOIL: 2-5 MIN
STEAM: 1-2 MIN
SAUTÉ: 1-2 MIN
OVEN ROAST: NOT RECOMMENDED
ON ITS OWN, BUT GREAT WHEN BAKED
WITH OTHER INGREDIENTS
(CASSEROLES, ARTICHOKE DIPS, ETC.)!

BOIL: 5-10 MIN
STEAM: 5-10 MIN
SAUTÉ: 3-5 MIN
OVEN ROAST: 450°F, 15 MIN

HOW TO BREW YOUR OWN ICED COFFEE

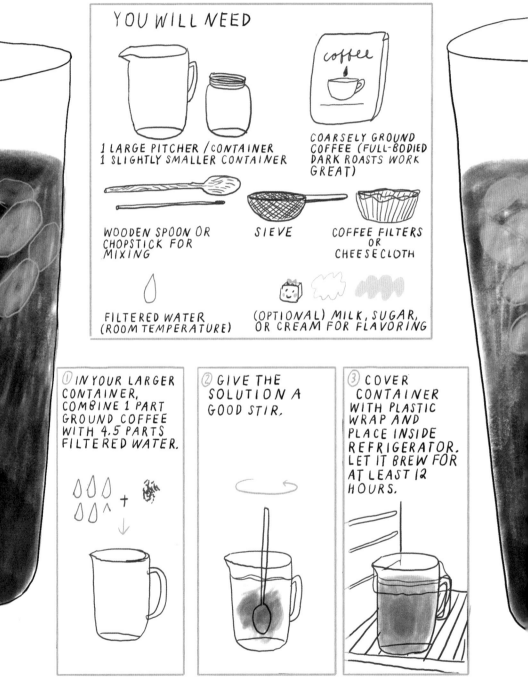

YOU WILL NEED

1 LARGE PITCHER / CONTAINER
1 SLIGHTLY SMALLER CONTAINER

COARSELY GROUND COFFEE (FULL-BODIED DARK ROASTS WORK GREAT)

WOODEN SPOON OR CHOPSTICK FOR MIXING

SIEVE

COFFEE FILTERS OR CHEESECLOTH

FILTERED WATER (ROOM TEMPERATURE)

(OPTIONAL) MILK, SUGAR, OR CREAM FOR FLAVORING

① IN YOUR LARGER CONTAINER, COMBINE 1 PART GROUND COFFEE WITH 4.5 PARTS FILTERED WATER.

② GIVE THE SOLUTION A GOOD STIR.

③ COVER CONTAINER WITH PLASTIC WRAP AND PLACE INSIDE REFRIGERATOR. LET IT BREW FOR AT LEAST 12 HOURS.

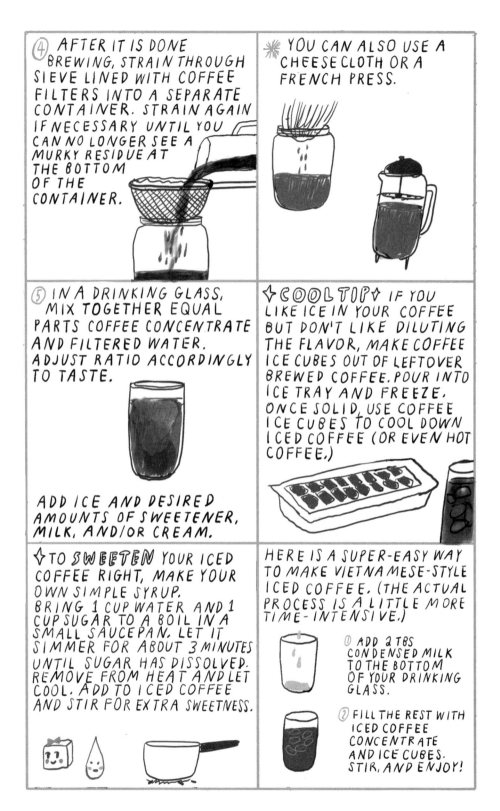

④ AFTER IT IS DONE BREWING, STRAIN THROUGH SIEVE LINED WITH COFFEE FILTERS INTO A SEPARATE CONTAINER. STRAIN AGAIN IF NECESSARY UNTIL YOU CAN NO LONGER SEE A MURKY RESIDUE AT THE BOTTOM OF THE CONTAINER.

✳ YOU CAN ALSO USE A CHEESECLOTH OR A FRENCH PRESS.

⑤ IN A DRINKING GLASS, MIX TOGETHER EQUAL PARTS COFFEE CONCENTRATE AND FILTERED WATER. ADJUST RATIO ACCORDINGLY TO TASTE.

ADD ICE AND DESIRED AMOUNTS OF SWEETENER, MILK, AND/OR CREAM.

✧COOL TIP✧ IF YOU LIKE ICE IN YOUR COFFEE BUT DON'T LIKE DILUTING THE FLAVOR, MAKE COFFEE ICE CUBES OUT OF LEFTOVER BREWED COFFEE. POUR INTO ICE TRAY AND FREEZE. ONCE SOLID, USE COFFEE ICE CUBES TO COOL DOWN ICED COFFEE (OR EVEN HOT COFFEE.)

✧TO SWEETEN YOUR ICED COFFEE RIGHT, MAKE YOUR OWN SIMPLE SYRUP. BRING 1 CUP WATER AND 1 CUP SUGAR TO A BOIL IN A SMALL SAUCEPAN. LET IT SIMMER FOR ABOUT 3 MINUTES UNTIL SUGAR HAS DISSOLVED. REMOVE FROM HEAT AND LET COOL. ADD TO ICED COFFEE AND STIR FOR EXTRA SWEETNESS.

HERE IS A SUPER-EASY WAY TO MAKE VIETNAMESE-STYLE ICED COFFEE. (THE ACTUAL PROCESS IS A LITTLE MORE TIME-INTENSIVE.)

① ADD 2 TBS CONDENSED MILK TO THE BOTTOM OF YOUR DRINKING GLASS.

② FILL THE REST WITH ICED COFFEE CONCENTRATE AND ICE CUBES. STIR, AND ENJOY!

HOW TO USE FRESH HERBS IN YOUR HOME COOKING

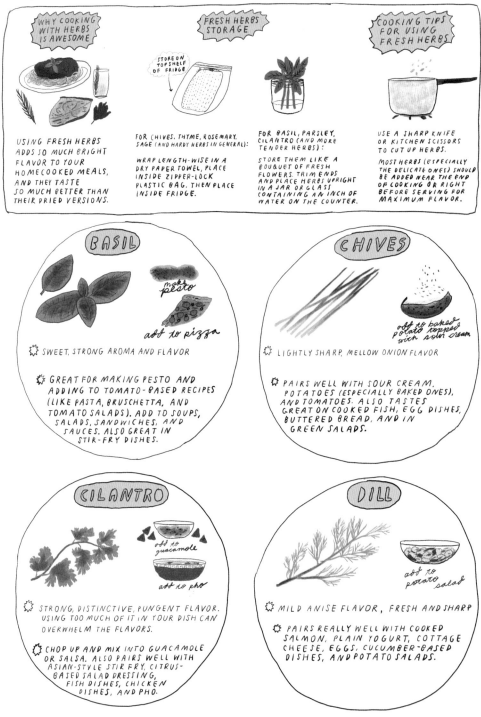

WHY COOKING WITH HERBS IS AWESOME

USING FRESH HERBS ADDS SO MUCH BRIGHT FLAVOR TO YOUR HOME COOKED MEALS, AND THEY TASTE SO MUCH BETTER THAN THEIR DRIED VERSIONS.

FRESH HERBS STORAGE

STORE ON TOP SHELF OF FRIDGE

FOR CHIVES. THYME, ROSEMARY, SAGE (AND HARDY HERBS IN GENERAL):

WRAP LENGTH-WISE IN A DRY PAPER TOWEL, PLACE INSIDE ZIPPER-LOCK PLASTIC BAG, THEN PLACE INSIDE FRIDGE.

FOR BASIL, PARSLEY, CILANTRO (AND MORE TENDER HERBS):

STORE THEM LIKE A BOUQUET OF FRESH FLOWERS. TRIM ENDS AND PLACE HERBS UPRIGHT IN A JAR OR GLASS CONTAINING AN INCH OF WATER ON THE COUNTER.

COOKING TIPS FOR USING FRESH HERBS

USE A SHARP KNIFE OR KITCHEN SCISSORS TO CUT UP HERBS.

MOST HERBS (ESPECIALLY THE DELICATE ONES) SHOULD BE ADDED NEAR THE END OF COOKING OR RIGHT BEFORE SERVING FOR MAXIMUM FLAVOR.

BASIL

make pesto

add to pizza

✿ SWEET, STRONG AROMA AND FLAVOR

✿ GREAT FOR MAKING PESTO AND ADDING TO TOMATO-BASED RECIPES (LIKE PASTA, BRUSCHETTA, AND TOMATO SALADS). ADD TO SOUPS, SALADS, SANDWICHES, AND SAUCES. ALSO GREAT IN STIR-FRY DISHES.

CHIVES

add to baked potato topped with sour cream

✿ LIGHTLY SHARP, MELLOW ONION FLAVOR

✿ PAIRS WELL WITH SOUR CREAM, POTATOES (ESPECIALLY BAKED ONES), AND TOMATOES. ALSO TASTES GREAT ON COOKED FISH, EGG DISHES, BUTTERED BREAD, AND IN GREEN SALADS.

CILANTRO

add to guacamole

add to pho

✿ STRONG, DISTINCTIVE, PUNGENT FLAVOR. USING TOO MUCH OF IT IN YOUR DISH CAN OVERWHELM THE FLAVORS.

✿ CHOP UP AND MIX INTO GUACAMOLE OR SALSA. ALSO PAIRS WELL WITH ASIAN-STYLE STIR FRY, CITRUS-BASED SALAD DRESSING, FISH DISHES, CHICKEN DISHES, AND PHO.

DILL

add to potato salad

✿ MILD ANISE FLAVOR, FRESH AND SHARP

✿ PAIRS REALLY WELL WITH COOKED SALMON, PLAIN YOGURT, COTTAGE CHEESE, EGGS, CUCUMBER-BASED DISHES, AND POTATO SALADS.

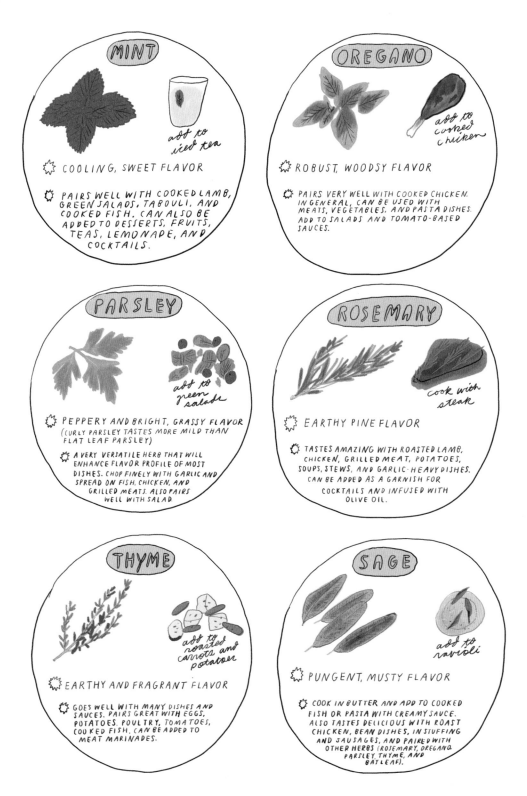

MINT

❋ COOLING, SWEET FLAVOR

✿ PAIRS WELL WITH COOKED LAMB, GREEN SALADS, TABOULI, AND COOKED FISH. CAN ALSO BE ADDED TO DESSERTS, FRUITS, TEAS, LEMONADE, AND COCKTAILS.

add to iced tea

OREGANO

❋ ROBUST, WOODSY FLAVOR

✿ PAIRS VERY WELL WITH COOKED CHICKEN. IN GENERAL, CAN BE USED WITH MEATS, VEGETABLES, AND PASTA DISHES. ADD TO SALADS AND TOMATO-BASED SAUCES.

add to cooked chicken

PARSLEY

❋ PEPPERY AND BRIGHT, GRASSY FLAVOR (CURLY PARSLEY TASTES MORE MILD THAN FLAT LEAF PARSLEY)

✿ A VERY VERSATILE HERB THAT WILL ENHANCE FLAVOR PROFILE OF MOST DISHES. CHOP FINELY WITH GARLIC AND SPREAD ON FISH, CHICKEN, AND GRILLED MEATS. ALSO PAIRS WELL WITH SALAD.

add to green salads

ROSEMARY

❋ EARTHY PINE FLAVOR

✿ TASTES AMAZING WITH ROASTED LAMB, CHICKEN, GRILLED MEAT, POTATOES, SOUPS, STEWS, AND GARLIC-HEAVY DISHES. CAN BE ADDED AS A GARNISH FOR COCKTAILS AND INFUSED WITH OLIVE OIL.

cook with steak

THYME

❋ EARTHY AND FRAGRANT FLAVOR

✿ GOES WELL WITH MANY DISHES AND SAUCES. PAIRS GREAT WITH EGGS, POTATOES, POULTRY, TOMATOES, COOKED FISH. CAN BE ADDED TO MEAT MARINADES.

add to roasted carrots and potatoes

SAGE

❋ PUNGENT, MUSTY FLAVOR

✿ COOK IN BUTTER AND ADD TO COOKED FISH OR PASTA WITH CREAMY SAUCE. ALSO TASTES DELICIOUS WITH ROAST CHICKEN, BEAN DISHES, IN STUFFING AND SAUSAGES, AND PAIRED WITH OTHER HERBS (ROSEMARY, OREGANO, PARSLEY, THYME, AND BAY LEAF).

add to ravioli

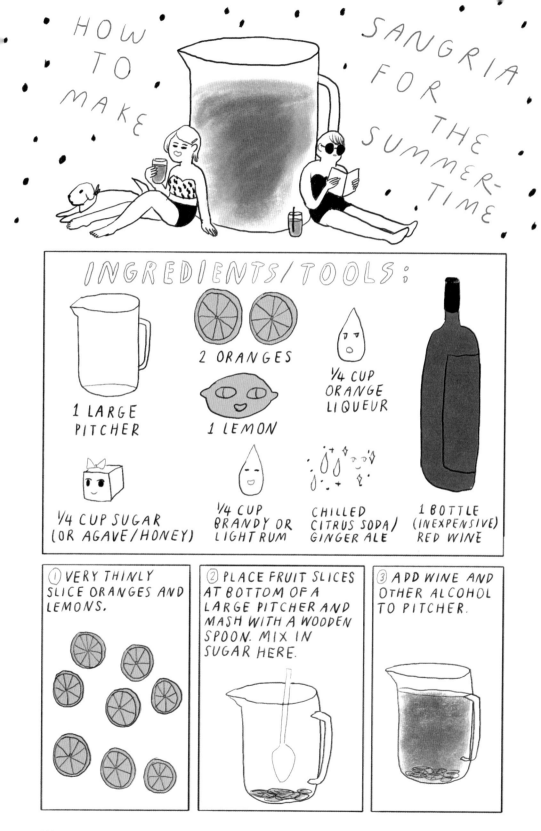

HOW TO MAKE SANGRIA FOR THE SUMMER-TIME

INGREDIENTS/TOOLS:

1 LARGE PITCHER

2 ORANGES

1 LEMON

¼ CUP ORANGE LIQUEUR

¼ CUP SUGAR (OR AGAVE/HONEY)

¼ CUP BRANDY OR LIGHT RUM

CHILLED CITRUS SODA/GINGER ALE

1 BOTTLE (INEXPENSIVE) RED WINE

① VERY THINLY SLICE ORANGES AND LEMONS.

② PLACE FRUIT SLICES AT BOTTOM OF A LARGE PITCHER AND MASH WITH A WOODEN SPOON. MIX IN SUGAR HERE.

③ ADD WINE AND OTHER ALCOHOL TO PITCHER.

④ COVER AND REFRIGERATE OVERNIGHT.

⑤ STRAIN OUT FRUIT. OR LEAVE THEM IN! IT'S UP TO YOU.

⑥ TO SERVE, POUR OVER ICE IN WINEGLASS AND ADD SODA TO TASTE.

⑦ YOU CAN ALSO ADD EXTRA GARNISHES LIKE FRESH MINT LEAVES, BASIL LEAVES, ROSEMARY, ETC.

❋ FOR AN EVEN FRUITIER SANGRIA, YOU CAN ADD MORE CHOPPED FRESH FRUIT (1-2 CUPS) LIKE APPLES, KIWI, BERRIES, WATERMELON, GRAPES, ETC.

SOAK THE FRUIT IN A SEPARATE SHALLOW CONTAINER OF RED WINE AND ADD TO EACH GLASS AS YOU SERVE.

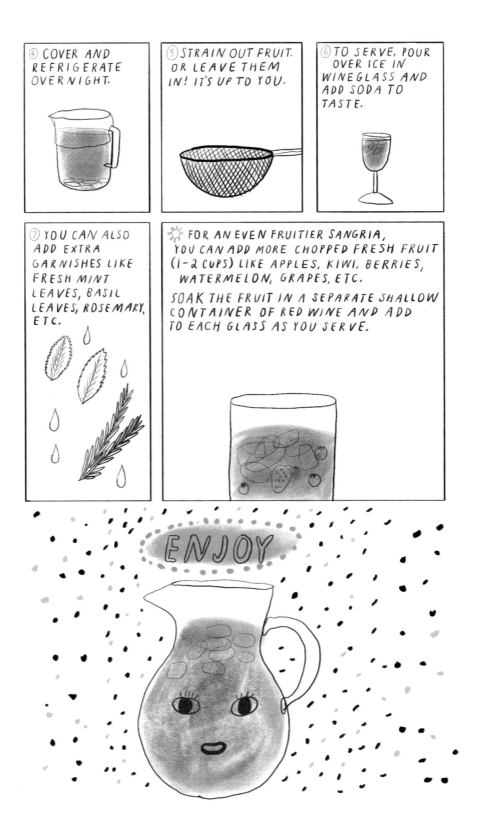

ENJOY

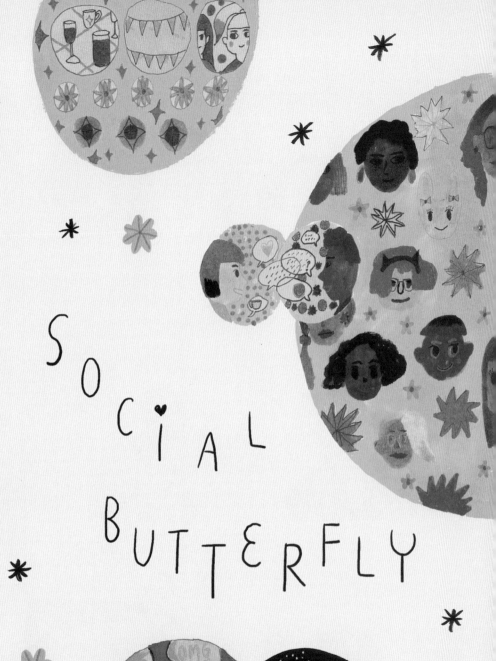

SOCIAL

BUTTERFLY

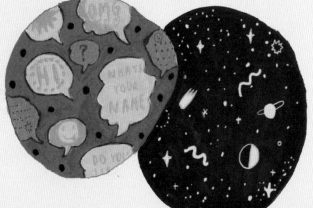

6 TRICKS TO HELP YOU REMEMBER PEOPLE'S NAMES AND FACES

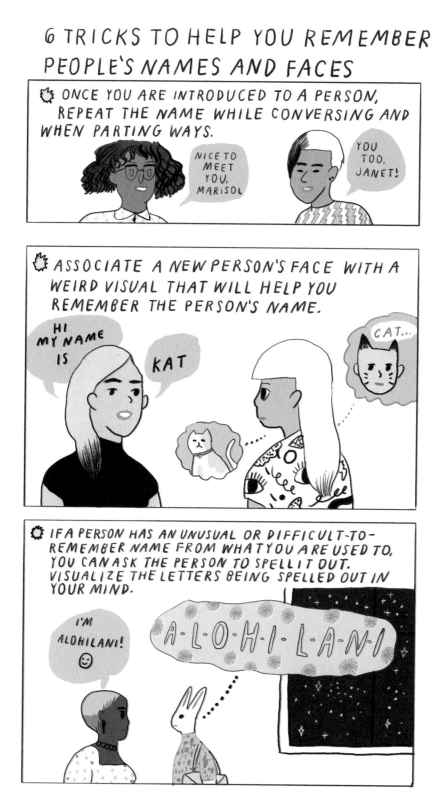

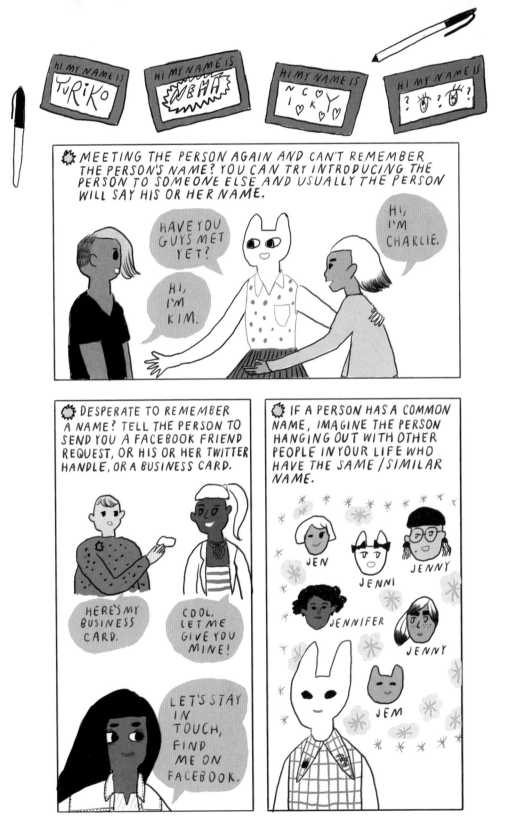

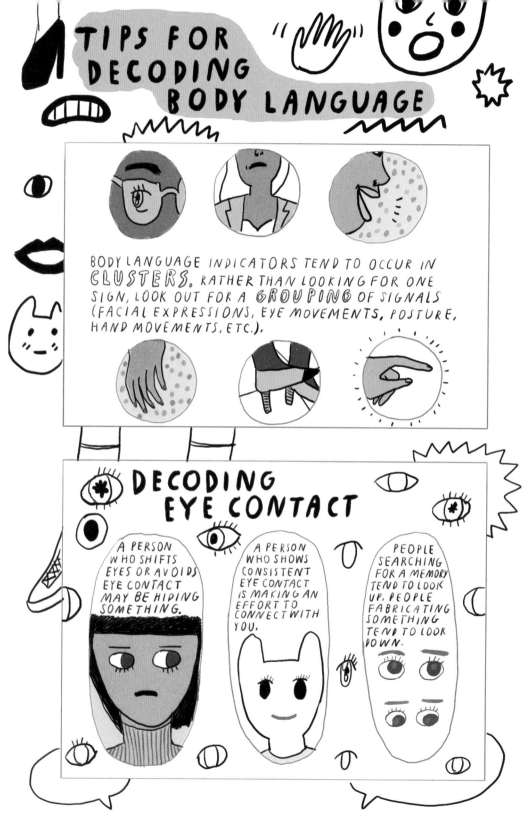

TIPS FOR DECODING BODY LANGUAGE

BODY LANGUAGE INDICATORS TEND TO OCCUR IN **CLUSTERS.** RATHER THAN LOOKING FOR ONE SIGN, LOOK OUT FOR A *GROUPING* OF SIGNALS (FACIAL EXPRESSIONS, EYE MOVEMENTS, POSTURE, HAND MOVEMENTS, ETC.).

DECODING EYE CONTACT

A PERSON WHO SHIFTS EYES OR AVOIDS EYE CONTACT MAY BE HIDING SOMETHING.

A PERSON WHO SHOWS CONSISTENT EYE CONTACT IS MAKING AN EFFORT TO CONNECT WITH YOU.

PEOPLE SEARCHING FOR A MEMORY TEND TO LOOK UP. PEOPLE FABRICATING SOMETHING TEND TO LOOK DOWN.

DECODING FACIAL EXPRESSION

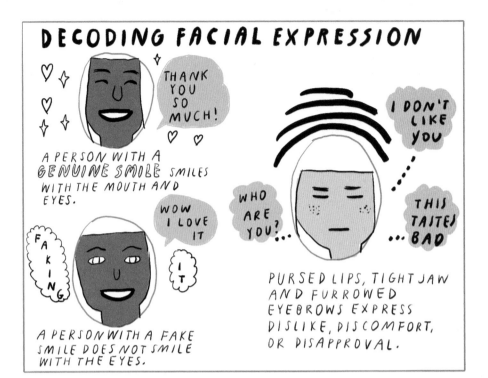

A PERSON WITH A GENUINE SMILE SMILES WITH THE MOUTH AND EYES.

A PERSON WITH A FAKE SMILE DOES NOT SMILE WITH THE EYES.

PURSED LIPS, TIGHT JAW AND FURROWED EYEBROWS EXPRESS DISLIKE, DISCOMFORT, OR DISAPPROVAL.

HOW CAN YOU TELL IF SOMEONE IS BORED? 3 SIGNS TO WATCH OUT FOR

① DISTRACTION
BORED PEOPLE TEND TO LOOK EVERYWHERE BUT THE PERSON SPEAKING TO THEM, THEY ALSO CAN BE CHECKING THE TIME OR LOOKING TOWARD AN EXIT.

② REPETITION
A BORED PERSON DOES REPETITIVE ACTIONS SUCH AS TAPPING FEET AND DRUMMING WITH FINGERS.

③ TIREDNESS
A BORED PERSON SLOUCHES OR SAGS, AND ACTS TIRED (LIKE EXCESSIVELY YAWNING).

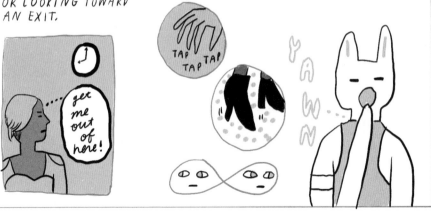

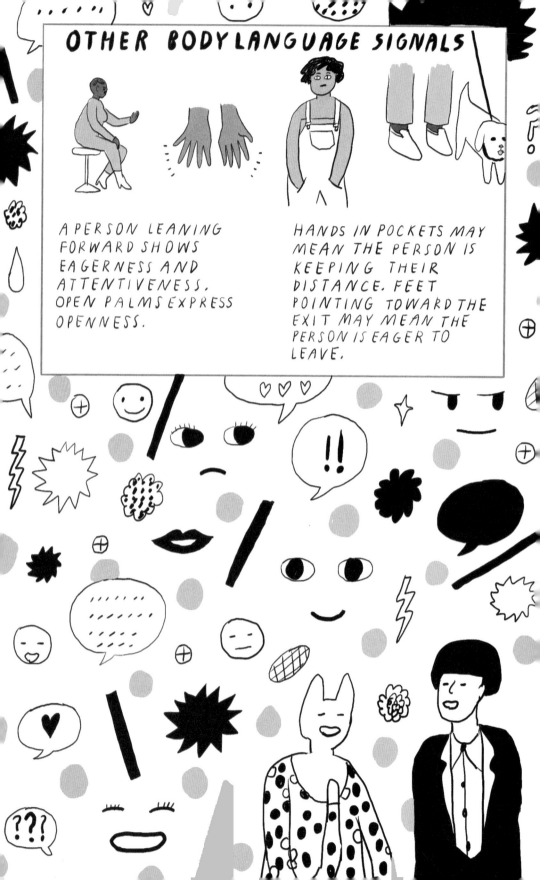

OTHER BODY LANGUAGE SIGNALS

A PERSON LEANING FORWARD SHOWS EAGERNESS AND ATTENTIVENESS. OPEN PALMS EXPRESS OPENNESS.

HANDS IN POCKETS MAY MEAN THE PERSON IS KEEPING THEIR DISTANCE. FEET POINTING TOWARD THE EXIT MAY MEAN THE PERSON IS EAGER TO LEAVE.

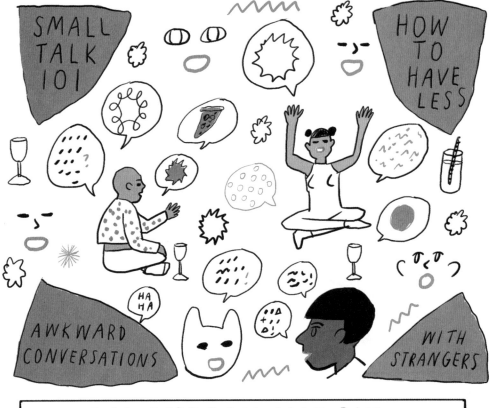

SMALL TALK 101

HOW TO HAVE LESS

AWKWARD CONVERSATIONS

WITH STRANGERS

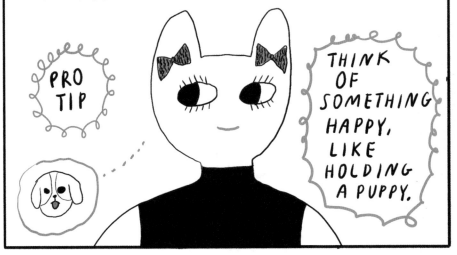

LOOK APPROACHABLE AND FRIENDLY. MAKE SURE YOU ARE WELL GROOMED / WELL DRESSED. MAKE A POINT TO LOOSEN YOUR FACIAL MUSCLES / SHOULDERS SO THAT YOU DON'T APPEAR TENSE.

PRO TIP

THINK OF SOMETHING HAPPY, LIKE HOLDING A PUPPY.

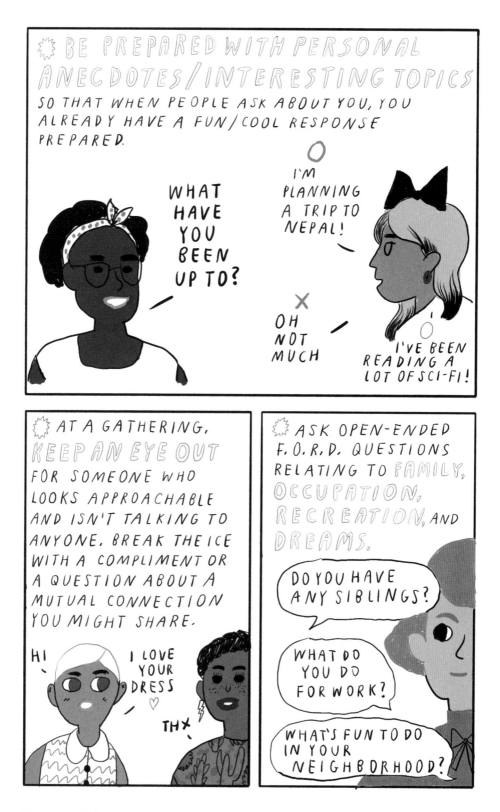

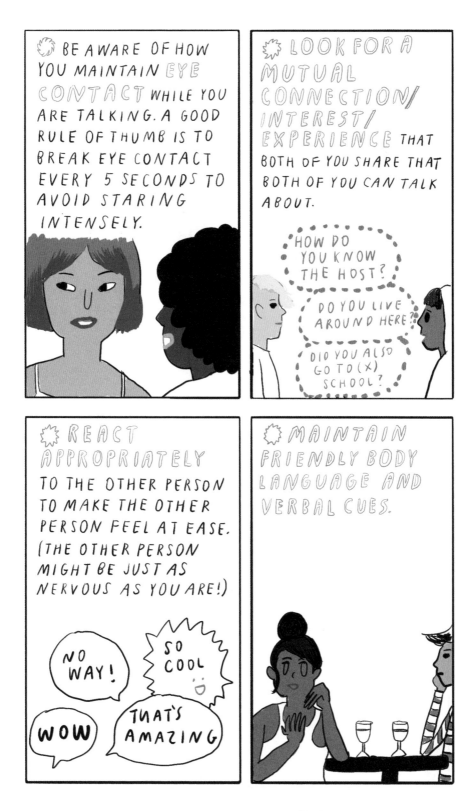

BE AWARE OF HOW YOU MAINTAIN EYE CONTACT WHILE YOU ARE TALKING. A GOOD RULE OF THUMB IS TO BREAK EYE CONTACT EVERY 5 SECONDS TO AVOID STARING INTENSELY.

LOOK FOR A MUTUAL CONNECTION/ INTEREST/ EXPERIENCE THAT BOTH OF YOU SHARE THAT BOTH OF YOU CAN TALK ABOUT.

HOW DO YOU KNOW THE HOST?

DO YOU LIVE AROUND HERE?

DID YOU ALSO GO TO (X) SCHOOL?

REACT APPROPRIATELY TO THE OTHER PERSON TO MAKE THE OTHER PERSON FEEL AT EASE. (THE OTHER PERSON MIGHT BE JUST AS NERVOUS AS YOU ARE!)

NO WAY!

SO COOL

WOW

THAT'S AMAZING

MAINTAIN FRIENDLY BODY LANGUAGE AND VERBAL CUES.

✻ **END ON A STRONG NOTE.** BE PREPARED WITH EXIT STRATEGIES SO THAT YOU CAN FINISH A CONVERSATION GRACEFULLY.

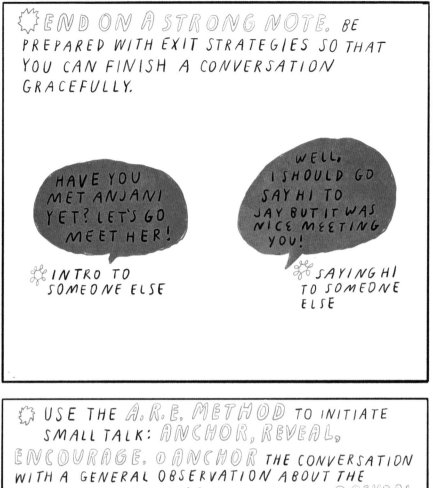

HAVE YOU MET ANJANI YET? LET'S GO MEET HER!

✻ INTRO TO SOMEONE ELSE

WELL, I SHOULD GO SAY HI TO JAY BUT IT WAS NICE MEETING YOU!

✻ SAYING HI TO SOMEONE ELSE

✻ USE THE *A.R.E. METHOD* TO INITIATE SMALL TALK: *ANCHOR, REVEAL, ENCOURAGE.* ① *ANCHOR* THE CONVERSATION WITH A GENERAL OBSERVATION ABOUT THE OCCASION YOU ARE BOTH A PART OF. ② *REVEAL* SOMETHING ABOUT YOURSELF, WHICH WILL THEN INVITE THE OTHER PERSON TO REVEAL SOMETHING, TOO. ③ *ENCOURAGE* THE CONVERSATION FURTHER BY ASKING OPEN-ENDED QUESTIONS THAT CAN'T BE ANSWERED WITH A YES / NO RESPONSE.

① ANCHOR

② REVEAL

③ ENCOURAGE

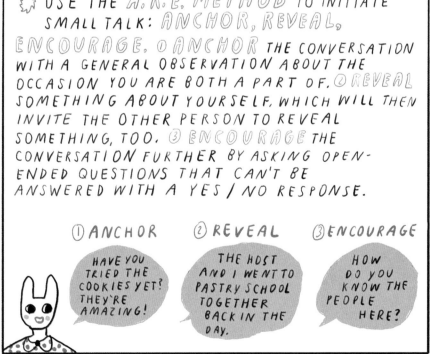

HAVE YOU TRIED THE COOKIES YET? THEY'RE AMAZING!

THE HOST AND I WENT TO PASTRY SCHOOL TOGETHER BACK IN THE DAY.

HOW DO YOU KNOW THE PEOPLE HERE?

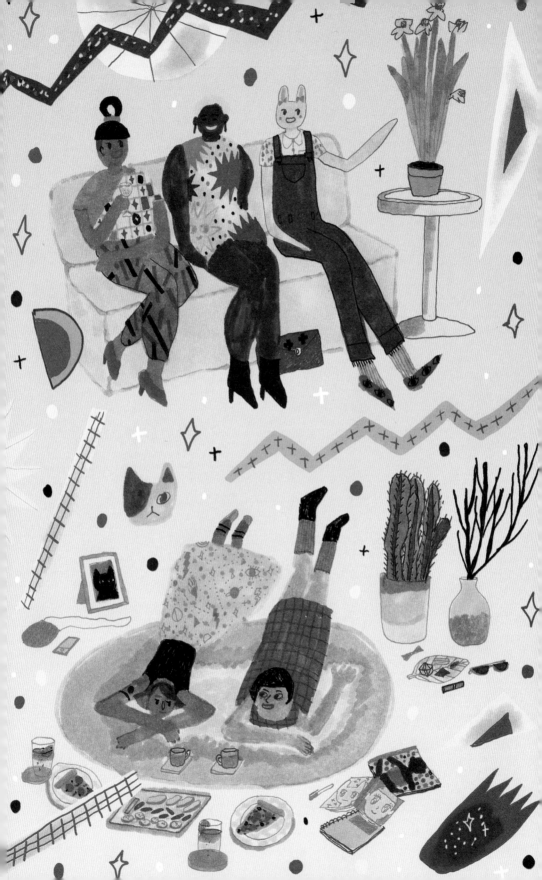

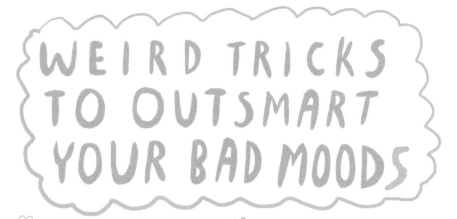

WEIRD TRICKS TO OUTSMART YOUR BAD MOODS

♡ SIT UP STRAIGHT, BREATHE DEEPLY, AND SMILE.

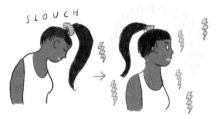

SOMETIMES WE FEEL A CERTAIN WAY BECAUSE OF HOW WE PHYSICALLY EXPRESS OURSELVES.

♡ EAT FOODS RICH IN FOLIC ACID.

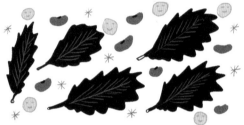

FOLIC ACID CAN LIFT YOUR SPIRITS. EAT A CUP OF BEANS OR A SALAD CONTAINING DARK, LEAFY GREENS.

♡ SNIFF A NOSTALGIC SMELL THAT MAKES YOU HAPPY.

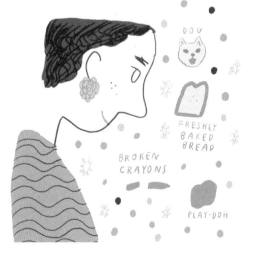

♡ SPEND $5 ON SOMEONE YOU CARE ABOUT.

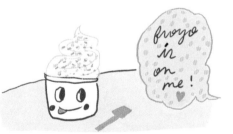

STUDIES HAVE SHOWN THAT PEOPLE WHO SPEND $ ON OTHERS FEEL WAY BETTER THAN PEOPLE WHO SPEND MONEY ON THEMSELVES.

♡ EAT A BAR OF DARK CHOCOLATE, WHICH HAS MOOD-BOOSTING PROPERTIES.

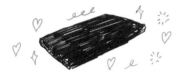

(SKIP THE SUGARY, MILK CHOCOLATE BLENDS.)

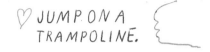

♡ JUMP ON A TRAMPOLINE.

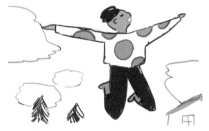

(OR IF YOU DON'T HAVE ACCESS TO A TRAMPOLINE, DO 10 JUMPING JACKS. PHYSICAL ACTIVITY = GREAT MOOD BOOST.)

♡ LOOK THROUGH A PHOTO ALBUM (ANALOG OR DIGITAL) TO REMIND YOURSELF OF HAPPY MOMENTS SPENT WITH LOVED ONES AND FRIENDS.

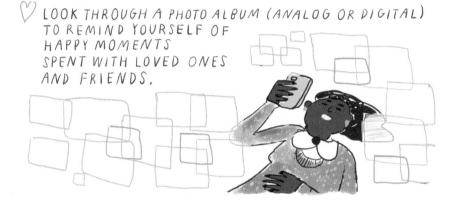

♡ THINK OF AN UPCOMING EVENT IN YOUR CALENDAR YOU ARE REALLY LOOKING FORWARD TO.

(OR SCHEDULE SOMETHING FUN FOR THE NEAR FUTURE!)

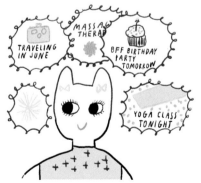

TRAVELING IN JUNE

MASSAGE THERAPY

BFF BIRTHDAY PARTY TOMORROW

YOGA CLASS TONIGHT

♡ SOMETIMES IT HELPS TO WRITE DOWN EVERYTHING THAT IS BOTHERING YOU AND IF APPLICABLE, WRITE DOWN A TANGIBLE SOLUTION FOR EACH PROBLEM.

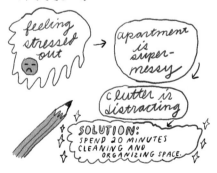

feeling stressed out → apartment is super-messy

clutter is distracting

SOLUTION: SPEND 20 MINUTES CLEANING AND ORGANIZING SPACE.

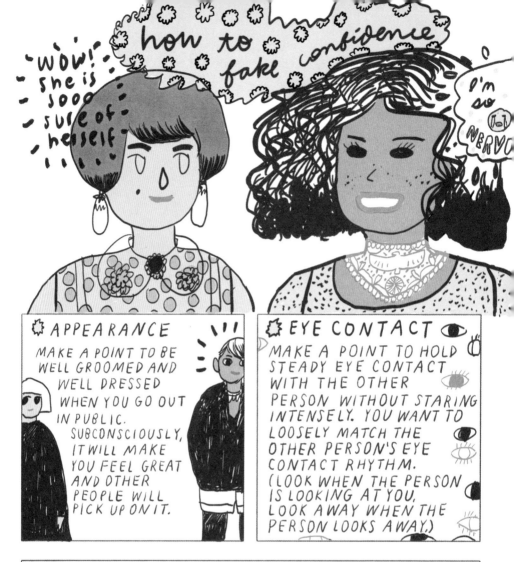

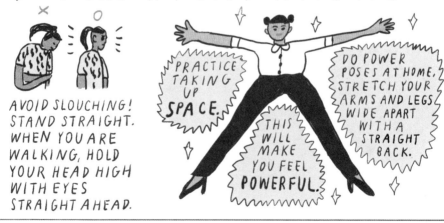

✺ SPEECH AND VERBAL LANGUAGE

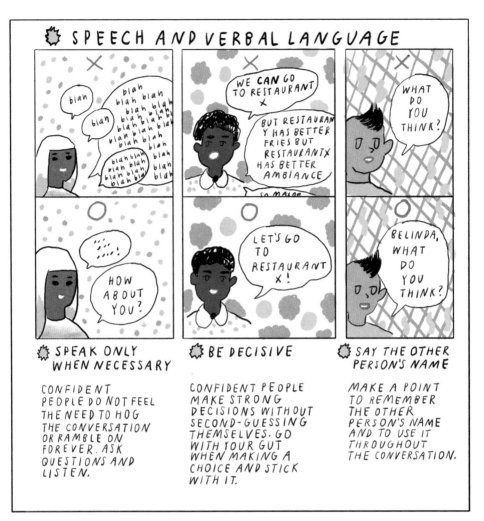

✺ SPEAK ONLY WHEN NECESSARY

CONFIDENT PEOPLE DO NOT FEEL THE NEED TO HOG THE CONVERSATION OR RAMBLE ON FOREVER. ASK QUESTIONS AND LISTEN.

✺ BE DECISIVE

CONFIDENT PEOPLE MAKE STRONG DECISIONS WITHOUT SECOND-GUESSING THEMSELVES. GO WITH YOUR GUT WHEN MAKING A CHOICE AND STICK WITH IT.

✺ SAY THE OTHER PERSON'S NAME

MAKE A POINT TO REMEMBER THE OTHER PERSON'S NAME AND TO USE IT THROUGHOUT THE CONVERSATION.

✺ ATTITUDE

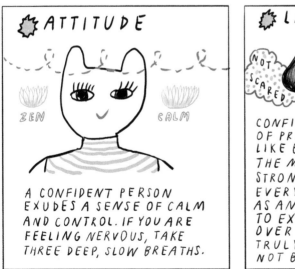

A CONFIDENT PERSON EXUDES A SENSE OF CALM AND CONTROL. IF YOU ARE FEELING NERVOUS, TAKE THREE DEEP, SLOW BREATHS.

✺ LAST...

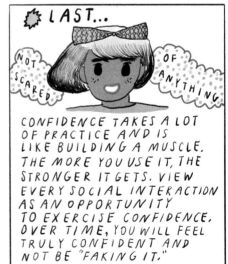

CONFIDENCE TAKES A LOT OF PRACTICE AND IS LIKE BUILDING A MUSCLE. THE MORE YOU USE IT, THE STRONGER IT GETS. VIEW EVERY SOCIAL INTERACTION AS AN OPPORTUNITY TO EXERCISE CONFIDENCE. OVER TIME, YOU WILL FEEL TRULY CONFIDENT AND NOT BE "FAKING IT."

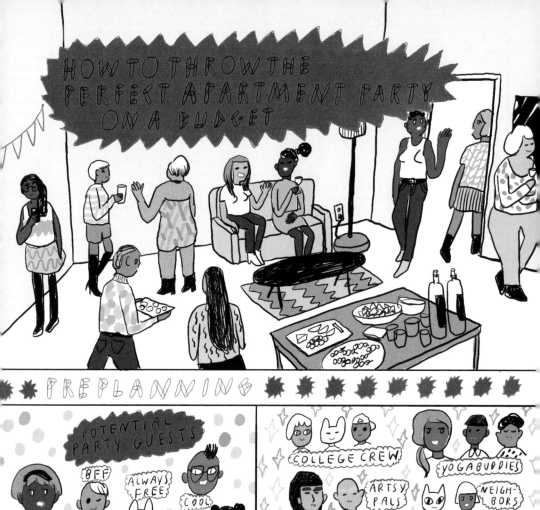

HOW TO THROW THE PERFECT APARTMENT PARTY ON A BUDGET

✳ PREPLANNING ✳ ✳ ✳ ✳ ✳ ✳ ✳ ✳ ✳

POTENTIAL PARTY GUESTS

LIFE OF PARTY
BFF
ALWAYS FREE
COOL
COUPLE
FLAKY
IN TOWN

COLLEGE CREW
YOGA BUDDIES
ARTSY PALS
NEIGHBORS

HAVE A REALISTIC IDEA OF HOW MANY PEOPLE WILL FIT COMFORTABLY INTO YOUR SPACE. TAKE INTO ACCOUNT +1'S, LAST-MINUTE CANCELLATIONS, BUSY SCHEDULES (ESPECIALLY IF IT IS HOLIDAY SEASON), ETC.

BE MINDFUL OF HOW ALL YOUR POTENTIAL PARTY GUESTS ARE GOING TO MINGLE WITH EACH OTHER. INVITE FRIENDS FROM DIFFERENT SOCIAL CIRCLES SO THE PARTY DOESN'T GET TOO CLIQUEY.

DEPENDING ON HOW CASUAL/UNCASUAL YOUR PARTY IS, SEND AN E-MAIL/SOCIAL MEDIA INVITE/PAPERLESS POST/PHYSICAL INVITATION A FEW WEEKS IN ADVANCE SO PEOPLE CAN PLAN AHEAD.

SUPER-EASY PARTY FOODS YOU CAN PREP AHEAD OF TIME

TIP FOOD PREPARED AHEAD OF TIME MEANS YOU CAN SPEND YOUR PARTY MINGLING WITH GUESTS INSTEAD OF BEING STUCK IN THE KITCHEN!

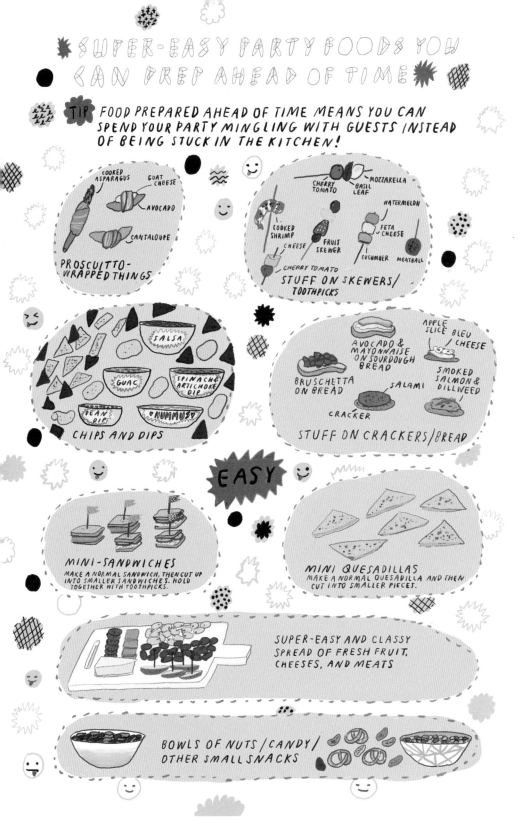

COOKED ASPARAGUS
GOAT CHEESE
AVOCADO
CANTALOUPE

PROSCUITTO-WRAPPED THINGS

CHERRY TOMATO
BASIL LEAF
MOZZARELLA
WATERMELON
COOKED SHRIMP
CHEESE
FRUIT SKEWER
FETA CHEESE
CUCUMBER
MEATBALL
CHERRY TOMATO

STUFF ON SKEWERS/ TOOTHPICKS

SALSA
GUAC
SPINACH & ARTICHOKE DIP
BEAN DIP
HUMMUS

CHIPS AND DIPS

AVOCADO & MAYONNAISE ON SOURDOUGH BREAD
APPLE SLICE
BLEU CHEESE
BRUSCHETTA ON BREAD
SALAMI
SMOKED SALMON & DILLWEED
CRACKER

STUFF ON CRACKERS/BREAD

EASY

MINI-SANDWICHES
MAKE A NORMAL SANDWICH, THEN CUT UP INTO SMALLER SANDWICHES. HOLD TOGETHER WITH TOOTHPICKS.

MINI QUESADILLAS
MAKE A NORMAL QUESADILLA AND THEN CUT INTO SMALLER PIECES.

SUPER-EASY AND CLASSY SPREAD OF FRESH FRUIT, CHEESES, AND MEATS

BOWLS OF NUTS/CANDY/ OTHER SMALL SNACKS

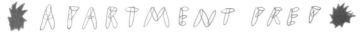

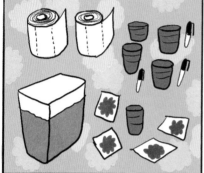

OPTIMIZE THE PEOPLE FLOW IN YOUR APARTMENT BY PUSHING FURNITURE AGAINST THE WALLS AND DECLUTTERING.

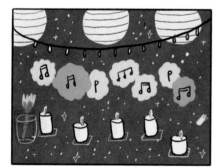

ANTICIPATE GUESTS' NEEDS. HAVE EXTRA TOILET PAPER ROLLS IN THE BATHROOM, EMPTY YOUR TRASH CAN, HAVE A CLEARLY MARKED RECYCLE AREA, SUPPLY SHARPIE PENS TO MARK NAMES ON PLASTIC CUPS, ETC.

MAKE LIGHTING DIM AND FLATTERING FOR THE GUESTS (NO HARSH OVERHEAD LIGHTING). EXTRA-FANCY TOUCH: HAVE A LIT TEALIGHT CANDLE IN THE BATHROOM, PLAY AMBIENT MUSIC IN THE BACKGROUND, TOO.

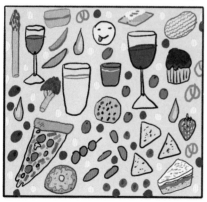

DON'T WORRY TOO MUCH ABOUT FOOD/DRINK! HAVE AN EMERGENCY BACKUP PLAN. YOU CAN ALWAYS ASK GUESTS/ FRIENDS TO CHIP IN WITH SNACKS/BYOB. (SEE NEXT GUIDE FOR PLANNING HOW MUCH FOOD AND DRINK TO PREPARE.)

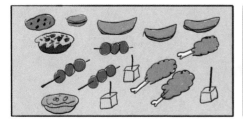

DON'T DEAL WITH FOODS THAT ARE COMPLICATED TO MAKE SO YOU ARE NOT STUCK ALL NIGHT IN THE KITCHEN.

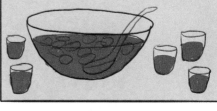

RATHER THAN MIXING DRINKS THROUGHOUT THE PARTY, HAVE 1-2 PRE-PREPARED PARTY DRINKS THAT GUESTS CAN HELP THEMSELVES TO.

✦ LET'S GET THE PARTY STARTED ✦

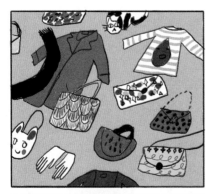

AS GUESTS ARRIVE, HAVE A DESIGNATED AREA FOR THEM TO LEAVE THEIR COATS, BAGS, AND PURSES (LIKE A SPARE ROOM OR YOUR BEDROOM).

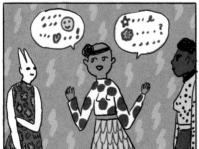

AS MUCH AS YOU CAN, INTRODUCE GUESTS TO ONE ANOTHER TO ENCOURAGE MINGLING OUTSIDE OF THEIR RESPECTIVE SOCIAL CIRCLES. GIVE A CONTEXT FOR HOW YOU KNOW EACH PERSON.

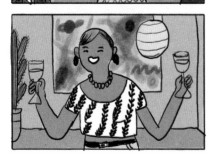

THROUGHOUT THE COURSE OF THE EVENING, BE ATTUNED TO YOUR GUESTS' NEEDS - LIKE IF SNACKS ARE RUNNING LOW, OR IF CERTAIN GUESTS NEED TO BE INTRODUCED TO MORE PEOPLE, ETC.

YOUR CHEAT SHEET FOR SERVING THE RIGHT AMOUNT OF FOOD AND DRINK AT A PARTY

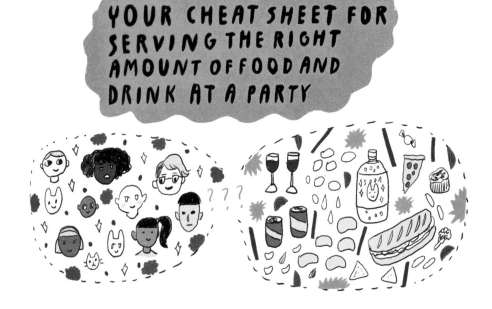

IN GENERAL....

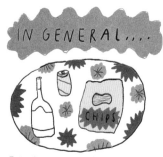

THESE GUIDELINES ARE NOT SET IN STONE! ULTIMATELY, GO WITH YOUR INSTINCTS.

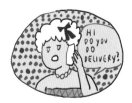

HAVE 1-2 BACKUP PLANS FOR THE WORST-CASE SCENARIO OF EVERYTHING RUNNING OUT.

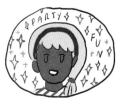

DON'T FREAK OUT! EVERYTHING IS GOING TO BE OKAY. ☺

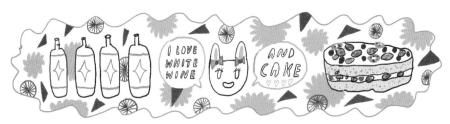

IF YOU PLAN ON INVESTING IN A LARGE QUANTITY OF FOOD AND DRINK, MAKE SURE IT IS FOOD AND DRINK YOU WOULD ACTUALLY ENJOY SHOULD YOU END UP WITH A LOT OF LEFTOVERS. (ALSO, MAYBE SOME GUESTS MIGHT WANT TO TAKE HOME LEFTOVER FOOD/DRINKS? HAVE EXTRA TO-GO CONTAINERS/TUPPERWARE ON HAND JUST IN CASE.)

FOOD AND DRINKS GUIDE FOR A COCKTAIL PARTY (NO DINNER)

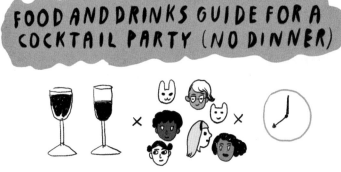

* 1.5 DRINKS PER HOUR PER GUEST.
(ADJUST ACCORDINGLY IF YOUR GUESTS ARE HEAVY DRINKERS, NONDRINKERS, ALL OF THE ABOVE, ETC.)

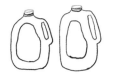 * ABOUT 2 GALLONS OF NONALCOHOLIC BEVERAGES FOR EVERY 25 GUESTS

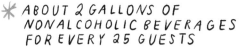

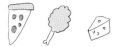 * 2 CUPS OF SNACKS PER PERSON

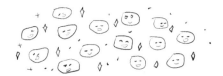 * ICE - FOR BIGGER PARTIES (ESPECIALLY OUTDOOR SUMMER PARTIES), PLAN ON 1lb PER PERSON. SMALLER - ABOUT 8 ICE CUBES PER PERSON

* 4-6 BITES OF FOOD PER PERSON PER HOUR

 * 1 SLICE OF CAKE OR 2 PIECES OF DESSERT PER PERSON

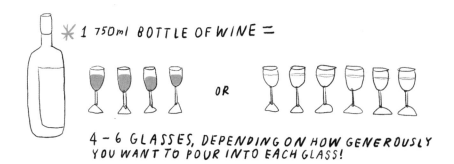

* 1 750ml BOTTLE OF WINE =

OR

4 - 6 GLASSES, DEPENDING ON HOW GENEROUSLY YOU WANT TO POUR INTO EACH GLASS!

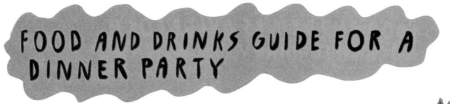

FOOD AND DRINKS GUIDE FOR A DINNER PARTY

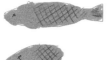

✳ MAIN ENTRÉE
1.5 SERVINGS
PER PERSON

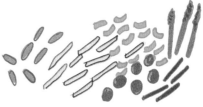

✳ SIDE DISH
2 CUPS
PER GUEST

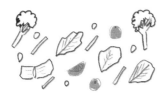

✳ SALAD
3-4 OZ PER
PERSON

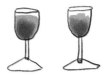

✳ WINE
2 GLASSES PER
GUEST

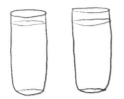

✳ NONALCOHOLIC BEVERAGE
2 16 OZ GLASSES
PER GUEST

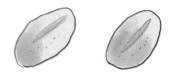

✳ BREAD/ROLLS
2 PIECES PER
PERSON

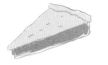

✳ DESSERT
1 PIECE/SLICE
PER PERSON

HAVE FUN

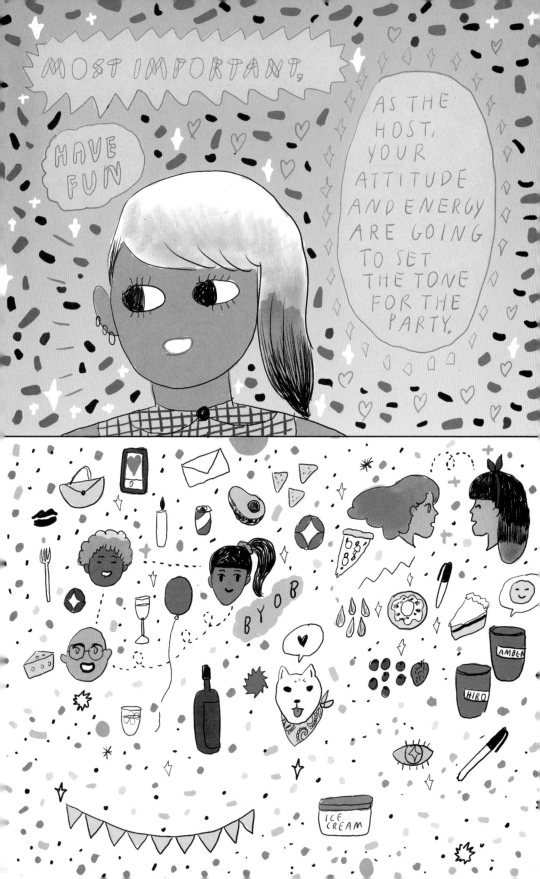

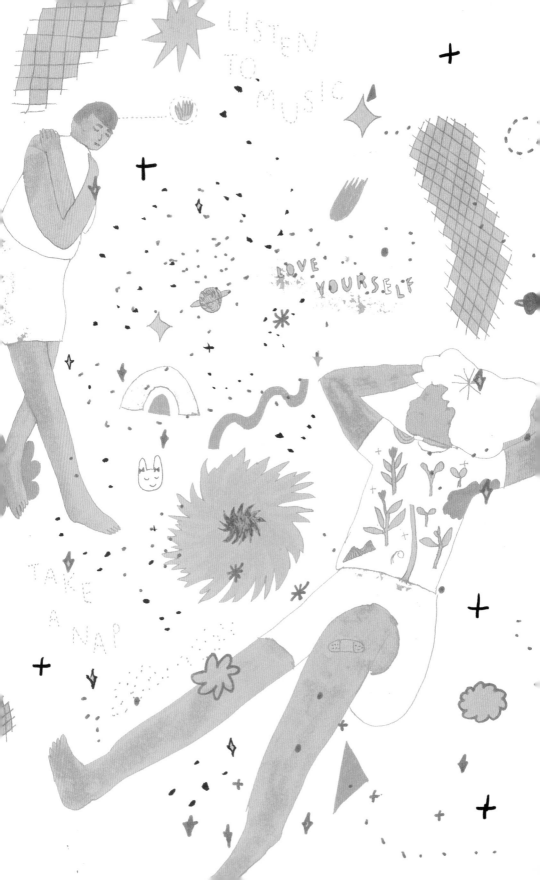

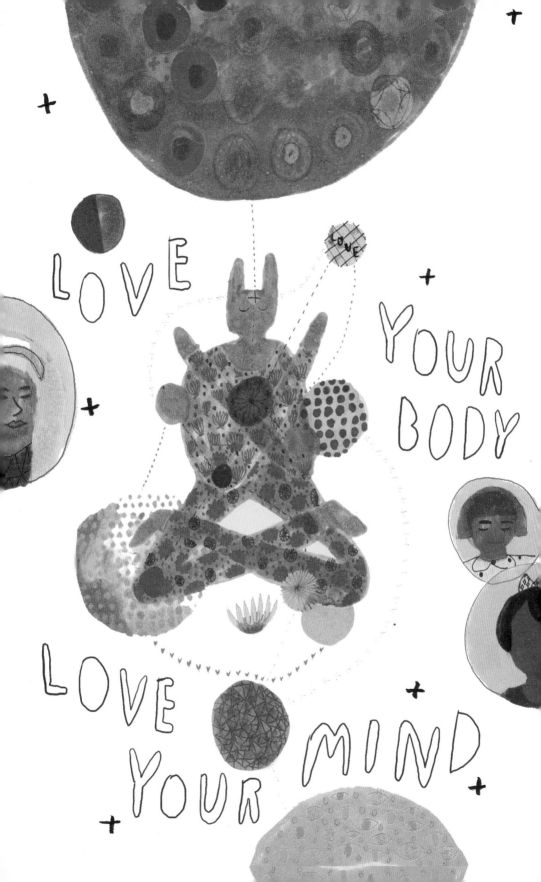

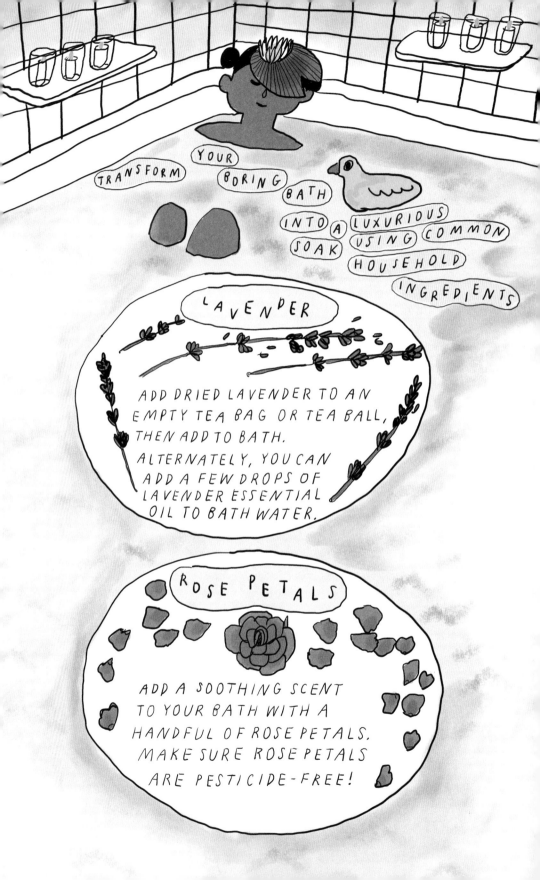

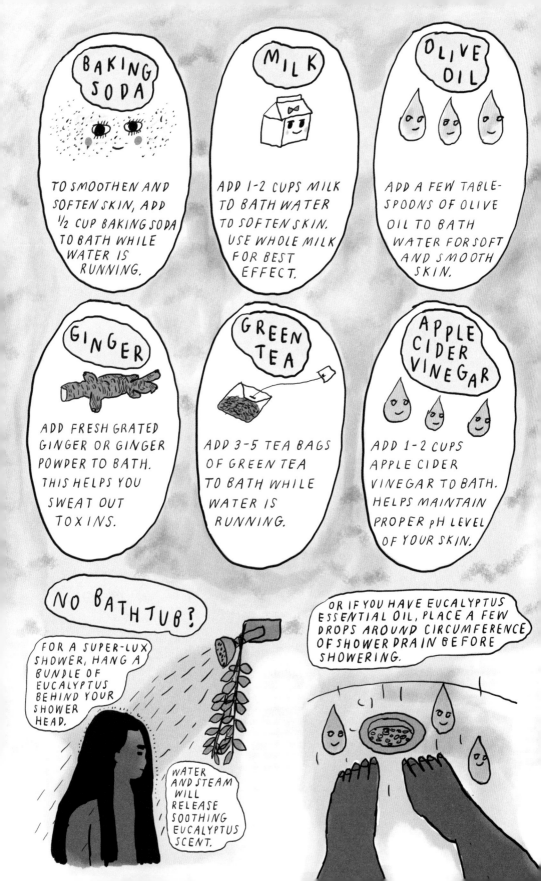

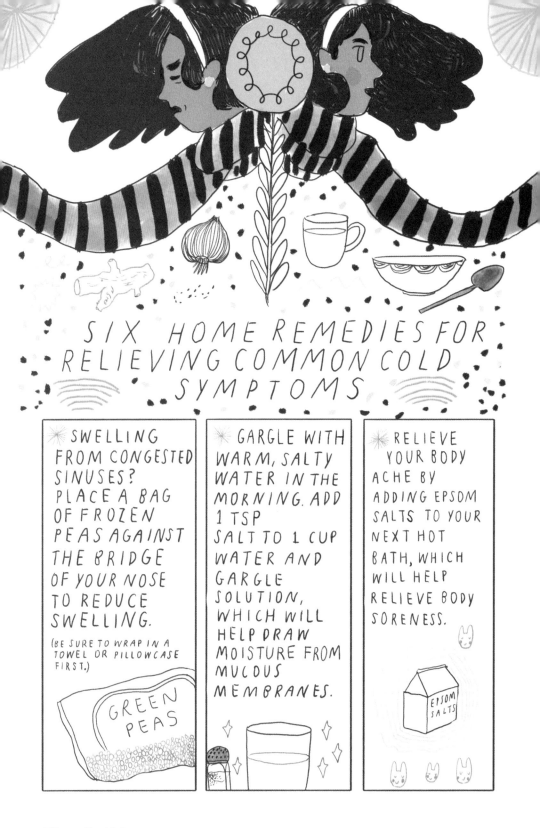

SIX HOME REMEDIES FOR RELIEVING COMMON COLD SYMPTOMS

SWELLING FROM CONGESTED SINUSES? PLACE A BAG OF FROZEN PEAS AGAINST THE BRIDGE OF YOUR NOSE TO REDUCE SWELLING.

(BE SURE TO WRAP IN A TOWEL OR PILLOWCASE FIRST.)

GREEN PEAS

GARGLE WITH WARM, SALTY WATER IN THE MORNING. ADD 1 TSP SALT TO 1 CUP WATER AND GARGLE SOLUTION, WHICH WILL HELP DRAW MOISTURE FROM MUCOUS MEMBRANES.

RELIEVE YOUR BODY ACHE BY ADDING EPSOM SALTS TO YOUR NEXT HOT BATH, WHICH WILL HELP RELIEVE BODY SORENESS.

EPSOM SALTS

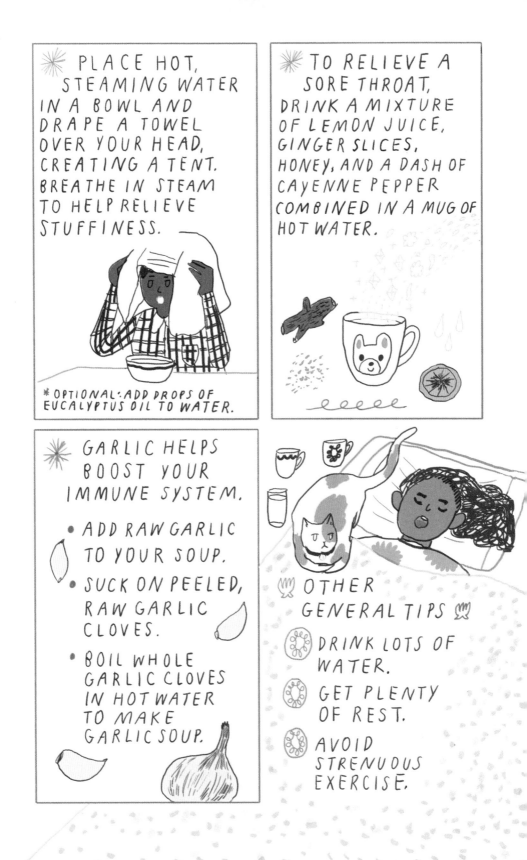

PLACE HOT, STEAMING WATER IN A BOWL AND DRAPE A TOWEL OVER YOUR HEAD, CREATING A TENT. BREATHE IN STEAM TO HELP RELIEVE STUFFINESS.

* OPTIONAL: ADD DROPS OF EUCALYPTUS OIL TO WATER.

TO RELIEVE A SORE THROAT, DRINK A MIXTURE OF LEMON JUICE, GINGER SLICES, HONEY, AND A DASH OF CAYENNE PEPPER COMBINED IN A MUG OF HOT WATER.

GARLIC HELPS BOOST YOUR IMMUNE SYSTEM.

- ADD RAW GARLIC TO YOUR SOUP.
- SUCK ON PEELED, RAW GARLIC CLOVES.
- BOIL WHOLE GARLIC CLOVES IN HOT WATER TO MAKE GARLIC SOUP.

OTHER GENERAL TIPS

DRINK LOTS OF WATER.

GET PLENTY OF REST.

AVOID STRENUOUS EXERCISE.

EASY BREATHING EXERCISES

CALMING DOWN

FOR

YOUR NERVES

SLOW AND STEADY BREATHS

one two three four five

one two three four five

exhale out

tension in chest

BODY SCAN

WE TEND TO TAKE SHORT, SHALLOW BREATHS WHEN WE FEEL STRESSED OUT. FOR A MORE CALMING EFFECT, INHALE DEEPLY THROUGH YOUR NOSE ON A SLOW COUNT OF FIVE AND EXHALE DEEPLY THROUGH YOUR MOUTH ON A SLOW COUNT OF FIVE. REPEAT FOR 5-10 CYCLES.

LIE DOWN IN A COMFORTABLE POSITION. DIRECT YOUR ATTENTION TO THE TOP OF YOUR HEAD ON YOUR INHALE. EXHALE OUT ANY TENSION YOU MAY BE FEELING. REPEAT THIS PROCESS FOR THE REST OF YOUR BODY, MOVING DOWNWARD FROM HEAD TO TOES. PAY EXTRA ATTENTION TO AREAS WHERE YOU FEEL THE MOST TENSION.

TIP!

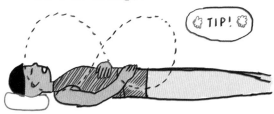

PLACE YOUR HAND ON YOUR STOMACH WHEN YOU ARE BREATHING. YOU SHOULD FEEL YOUR STOMACH EXPAND WHEN YOU INHALE AND CONTRACT WHEN YOU EXHALE.

ALTERNATIVE NOSTRIL BREATH

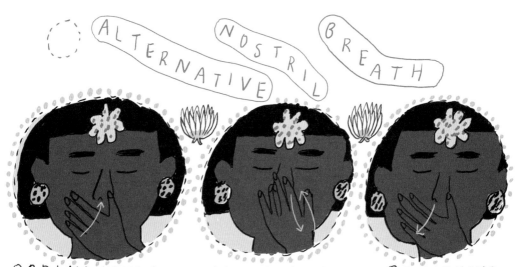

① BRING YOUR RIGHT HAND TO YOUR FACE. ② PLACE YOUR RIGHT THUMB OVER YOUR RIGHT NOSTRIL, INHALE SLOWLY THROUGH YOUR LEFT NOSTRIL. ③ CLOSE YOUR LEFT NOSTRIL WITH YOUR RING FINGER AND RELEASE THUMB FROM YOUR RIGHT NOSTRIL. ④ EXHALE THROUGH YOUR RIGHT NOSTRIL. ⑤ INHALE THROUGH YOUR RIGHT NOSTRIL. ⑥ CLOSE YOUR RIGHT NOSTRIL WITH YOUR RIGHT THUMB AND RELEASE RING FINGER FROM YOUR LEFT NOSTRIL. ⑦ EXHALE THROUGH YOUR LEFT NOSTRIL. REPEAT CYCLE FOR 3-5 MINUTES.

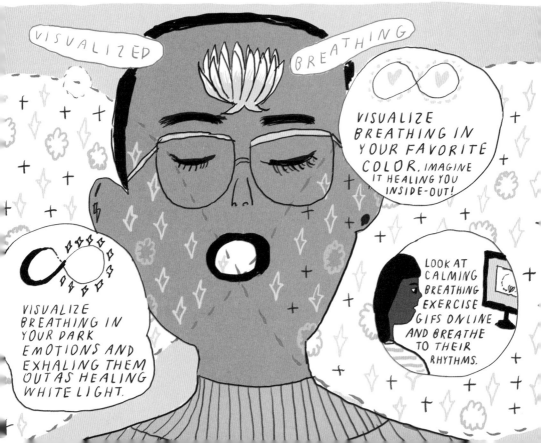

VISUALIZED BREATHING

VISUALIZE BREATHING IN YOUR FAVORITE COLOR. IMAGINE IT HEALING YOU INSIDE-OUT!

VISUALIZE BREATHING IN YOUR DARK EMOTIONS AND EXHALING THEM OUT AS HEALING WHITE LIGHT.

LOOK AT CALMING BREATHING EXERCISE GIFS ONLINE AND BREATHE TO THEIR RHYTHMS.

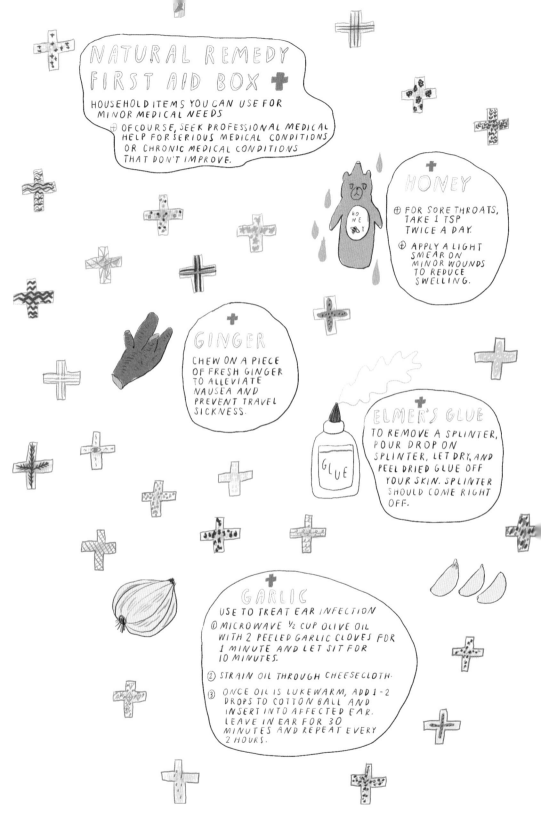

NATURAL REMEDY FIRST AID BOX ✚

HOUSEHOLD ITEMS YOU CAN USE FOR MINOR MEDICAL NEEDS

⊕ OF COURSE, SEEK PROFESSIONAL MEDICAL HELP FOR SERIOUS MEDICAL CONDITIONS OR CHRONIC MEDICAL CONDITIONS THAT DON'T IMPROVE.

HONEY

⊕ FOR SORE THROATS, TAKE 1 TSP TWICE A DAY.

⊕ APPLY A LIGHT SMEAR ON MINOR WOUNDS TO REDUCE SWELLING.

GINGER

CHEW ON A PIECE OF FRESH GINGER TO ALLEVIATE NAUSEA AND PREVENT TRAVEL SICKNESS.

ELMER'S GLUE

TO REMOVE A SPLINTER, POUR DROP ON SPLINTER, LET DRY, AND PEEL DRIED GLUE OFF YOUR SKIN. SPLINTER SHOULD COME RIGHT OFF.

GARLIC

USE TO TREAT EAR INFECTION

① MICROWAVE ½ CUP OLIVE OIL WITH 2 PEELED GARLIC CLOVES FOR 1 MINUTE AND LET SIT FOR 10 MINUTES.

② STRAIN OIL THROUGH CHEESECLOTH.

③ ONCE OIL IS LUKEWARM, ADD 1-2 DROPS TO COTTON BALL AND INSERT INTO AFFECTED EAR. LEAVE IN EAR FOR 30 MINUTES AND REPEAT EVERY 2 HOURS.

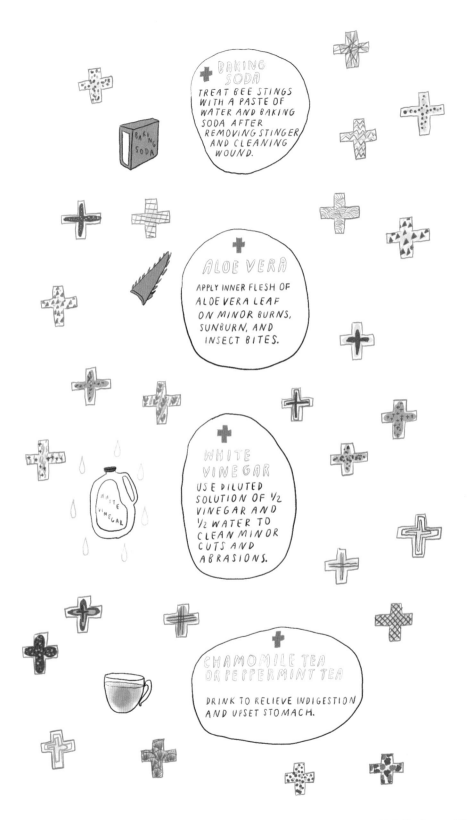

BAKING SODA
TREAT BEE STINGS WITH A PASTE OF WATER AND BAKING SODA AFTER REMOVING STINGER AND CLEANING WOUND.

ALOE VERA
APPLY INNER FLESH OF ALOE VERA LEAF ON MINOR BURNS, SUNBURN, AND INSECT BITES.

WHITE VINEGAR
USE DILUTED SOLUTION OF ½ VINEGAR AND ½ WATER TO CLEAN MINOR CUTS AND ABRASIONS.

CHAMOMILE TEA OR PEPPERMINT TEA
DRINK TO RELIEVE INDIGESTION AND UPSET STOMACH.

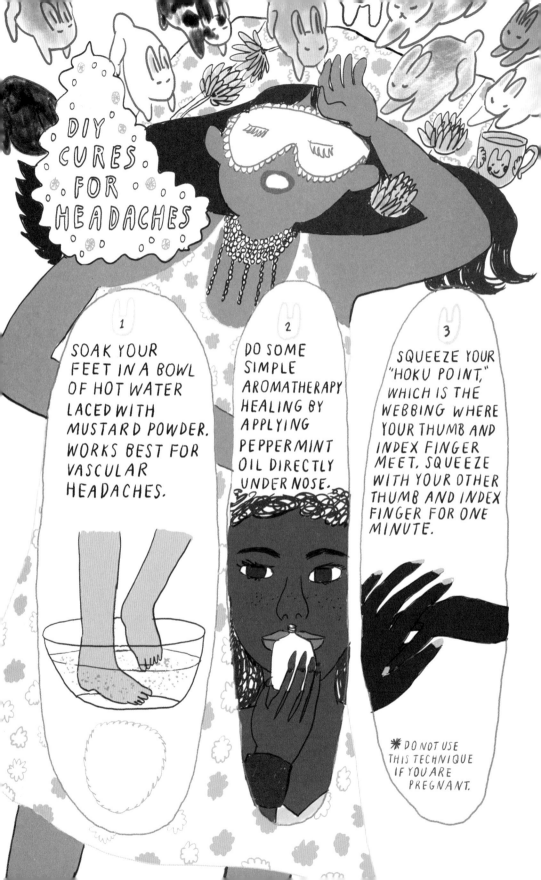

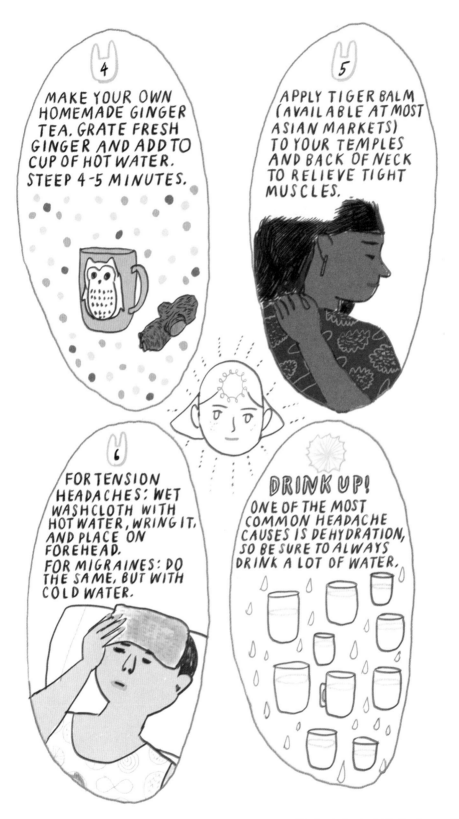

4

MAKE YOUR OWN HOMEMADE GINGER TEA. GRATE FRESH GINGER AND ADD TO CUP OF HOT WATER. STEEP 4-5 MINUTES.

5

APPLY TIGER BALM (AVAILABLE AT MOST ASIAN MARKETS) TO YOUR TEMPLES AND BACK OF NECK TO RELIEVE TIGHT MUSCLES.

6

FOR TENSION HEADACHES: WET WASHCLOTH WITH HOT WATER, WRING IT, AND PLACE ON FOREHEAD. FOR MIGRAINES: DO THE SAME, BUT WITH COLD WATER.

DRINK UP!
ONE OF THE MOST COMMON HEADACHE CAUSES IS DEHYDRATION, SO BE SURE TO ALWAYS DRINK A LOT OF WATER.

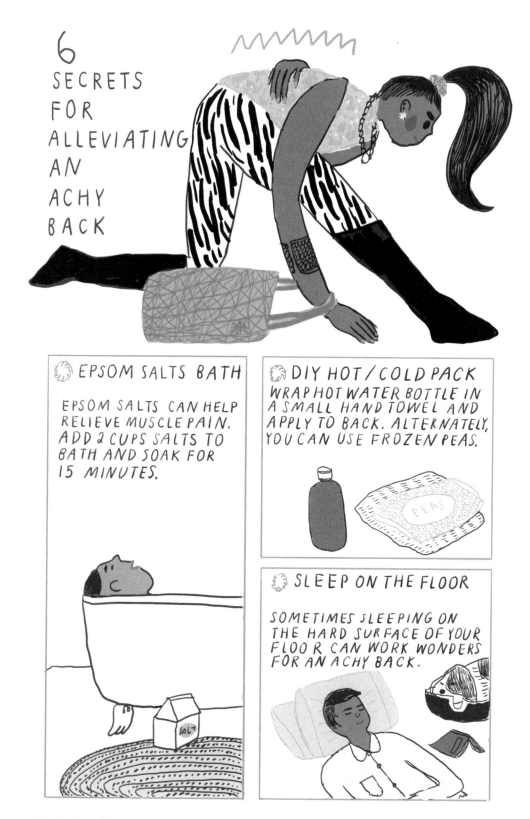

6 SECRETS FOR ALLEVIATING AN ACHY BACK

EPSOM SALTS BATH

EPSOM SALTS CAN HELP RELIEVE MUSCLE PAIN. ADD 2 CUPS SALTS TO BATH AND SOAK FOR 15 MINUTES.

DIY HOT/COLD PACK

WRAP HOT WATER BOTTLE IN A SMALL HAND TOWEL AND APPLY TO BACK. ALTERNATELY, YOU CAN USE FROZEN PEAS.

PEAS

SLEEP ON THE FLOOR

SOMETIMES SLEEPING ON THE HARD SURFACE OF YOUR FLOOR CAN WORK WONDERS FOR AN ACHY BACK.

TENNIS BALLS IN SOCK

PLACE 2 TENNIS BALLS IN A LONG SOCK AND TIE END. PLACE ON FLOOR AND ROLL ON IT WITH YOUR BACK, OR PLACE BALLS BETWEEN YOUR BACK AND A WALL WHILE SITTING IN THE AIR UPRIGHT.

ACUPRESSURE MAT

AVAILABLE ONLINE OR AT SPECIALIZED HEALTH STORES, ACUPRESSURE MATS CAN HELP RELIEVE CHRONIC BACK PAIN OR SORENESS. REST ON MAT FOR 30 MINUTES BEFORE GOING TO BED OR IN THE MORNING AFTER WAKING UP.

YOGA

PRACTICING YOGA CAN HELP EASE LOWER BACK PAIN. A FEW SIMPLE BEGINNER'S POSES YOU CAN DO:

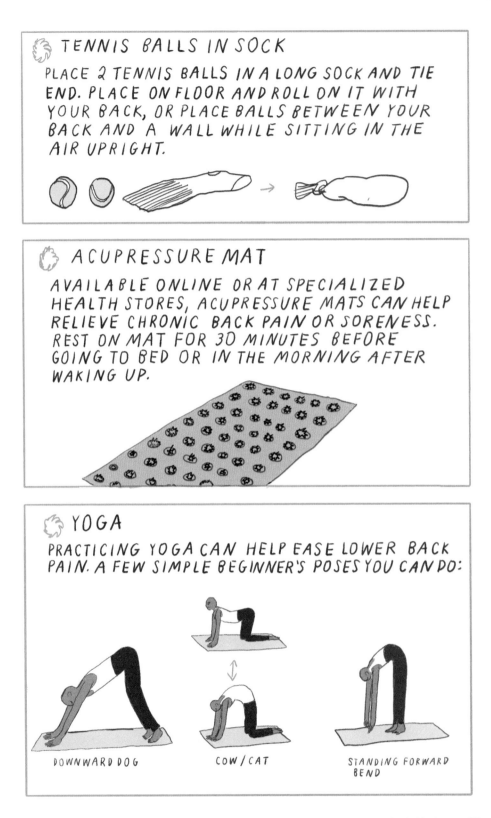

DOWNWARD DOG

COW / CAT

STANDING FORWARD BEND

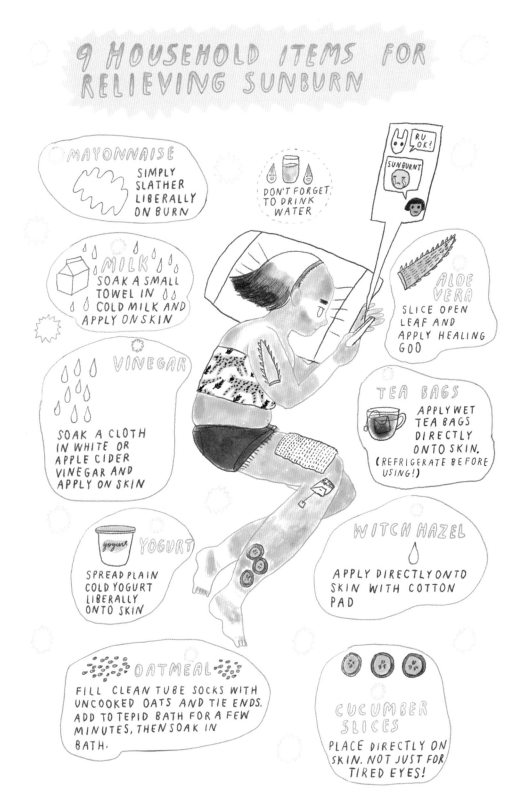

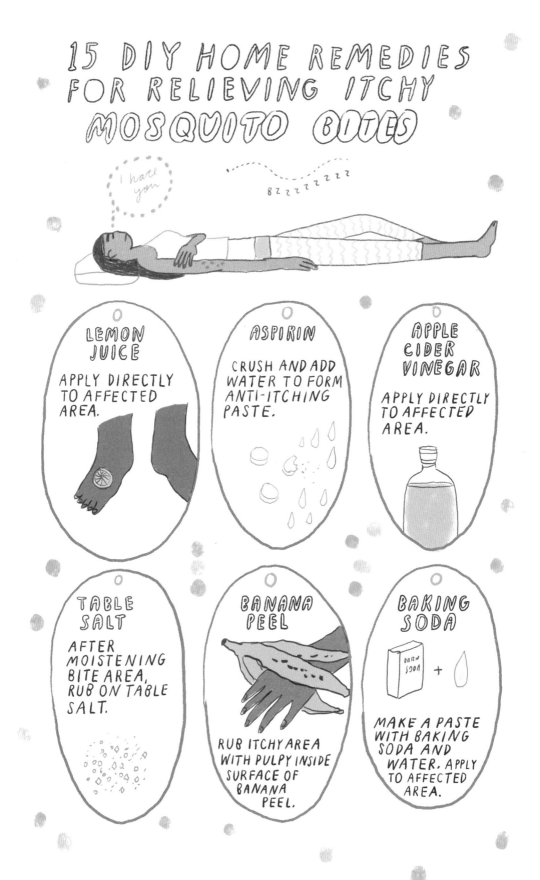

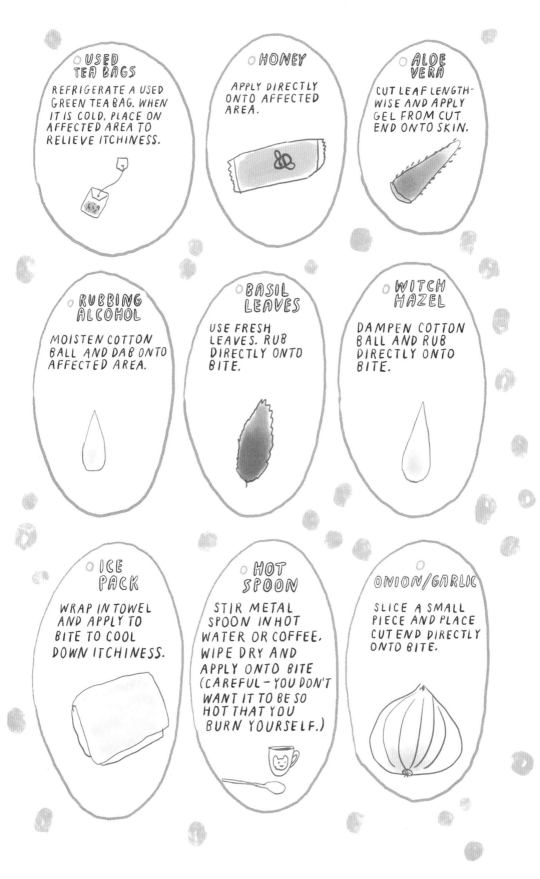

USED TEA BAGS
REFRIGERATE A USED GREEN TEA BAG. WHEN IT IS COLD, PLACE ON AFFECTED AREA TO RELIEVE ITCHINESS.

HONEY
APPLY DIRECTLY ONTO AFFECTED AREA.

ALOE VERA
CUT LEAF LENGTHWISE AND APPLY GEL FROM CUT END ONTO SKIN.

RUBBING ALCOHOL
MOISTEN COTTON BALL AND DAB ONTO AFFECTED AREA.

BASIL LEAVES
USE FRESH LEAVES. RUB DIRECTLY ONTO BITE.

WITCH HAZEL
DAMPEN COTTON BALL AND RUB DIRECTLY ONTO BITE.

ICE PACK
WRAP IN TOWEL AND APPLY TO BITE TO COOL DOWN ITCHINESS.

HOT SPOON
STIR METAL SPOON IN HOT WATER OR COFFEE. WIPE DRY AND APPLY ONTO BITE (CAREFUL — YOU DON'T WANT IT TO BE SO HOT THAT YOU BURN YOURSELF.)

ONION/GARLIC
SLICE A SMALL PIECE AND PLACE CUT END DIRECTLY ONTO BITE.

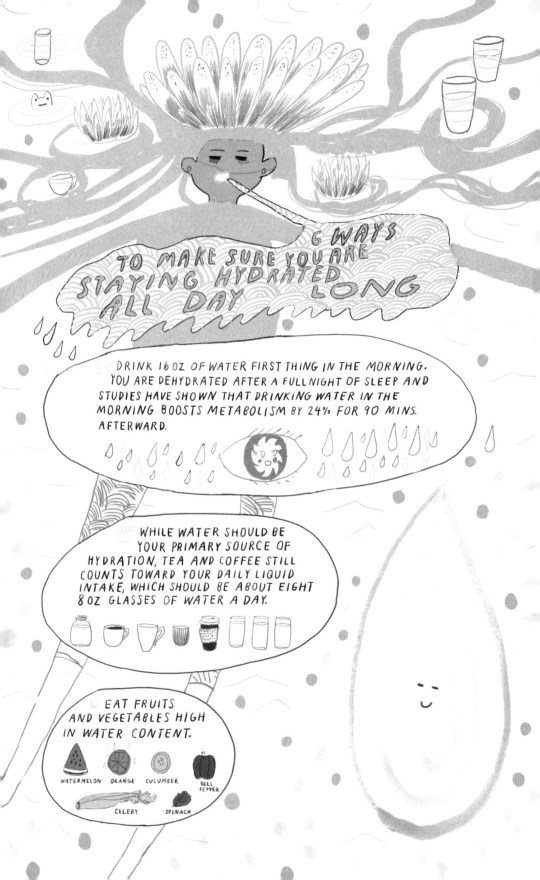

6 WAYS TO MAKE SURE YOU ARE STAYING HYDRATED ALL DAY LONG

DRINK 16 OZ OF WATER FIRST THING IN THE MORNING. YOU ARE DEHYDRATED AFTER A FULL NIGHT OF SLEEP AND STUDIES HAVE SHOWN THAT DRINKING WATER IN THE MORNING BOOSTS METABOLISM BY 24% FOR 90 MINS. AFTERWARD.

WHILE WATER SHOULD BE YOUR PRIMARY SOURCE OF HYDRATION, TEA AND COFFEE STILL COUNTS TOWARD YOUR DAILY LIQUID INTAKE, WHICH SHOULD BE ABOUT EIGHT 8 OZ GLASSES OF WATER A DAY.

EAT FRUITS AND VEGETABLES HIGH IN WATER CONTENT.

WATERMELON   ORANGE   CUCUMBER   BELL PEPPER

CELERY   SPINACH

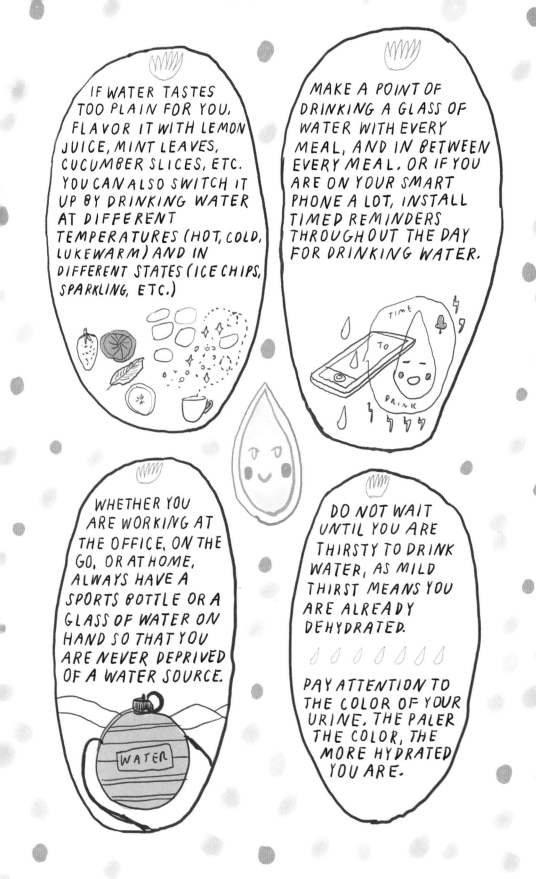

IF WATER TASTES TOO PLAIN FOR YOU, FLAVOR IT WITH LEMON JUICE, MINT LEAVES, CUCUMBER SLICES, ETC. YOU CAN ALSO SWITCH IT UP BY DRINKING WATER AT DIFFERENT TEMPERATURES (HOT, COLD, LUKEWARM) AND IN DIFFERENT STATES (ICE CHIPS, SPARKLING, ETC.)

MAKE A POINT OF DRINKING A GLASS OF WATER WITH EVERY MEAL, AND IN BETWEEN EVERY MEAL. OR IF YOU ARE ON YOUR SMART PHONE A LOT, INSTALL TIMED REMINDERS THROUGHOUT THE DAY FOR DRINKING WATER.

TIME TO DRINK

WHETHER YOU ARE WORKING AT THE OFFICE, ON THE GO, OR AT HOME, ALWAYS HAVE A SPORTS BOTTLE OR A GLASS OF WATER ON HAND SO THAT YOU ARE NEVER DEPRIVED OF A WATER SOURCE.

WATER

DO NOT WAIT UNTIL YOU ARE THIRSTY TO DRINK WATER, AS MILD THIRST MEANS YOU ARE ALREADY DEHYDRATED.

PAY ATTENTION TO THE COLOR OF YOUR URINE. THE PALER THE COLOR, THE MORE HYDRATED YOU ARE.

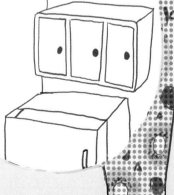

13 TRICKS FOR

EATING HEALTHIER

EAT THE HEALTHIEST FOOD ON YOUR PLATE FIRST (OR WHATEVER IS IN FRONT OF YOU). THIS WAY, YOU WILL BE LESS LIKELY TO BINGE ON UNHEALTHY ITEMS.

TO SUPPRESS YOUR APPETITE, SNIFF A BANANA OR AN APPLE. TO SUPPRESS SWEET CRAVINGS, SNIFF SOMETHING VANILLA-SCENTED.

SNIFF

PLACE INDULGENT FOODS IN HARD-TO-REACH/OUT-OF-SIGHT PLACES.

KEEP A FOOD JOURNAL. BY WRITING DOWN WHAT YOU EAT AND HOW IT AFFECTS YOU (MENTALLY AND PHYSICALLY), YOU WILL MAKE MORE MINDFUL CHOICES REGARDING WHAT YOU EAT.

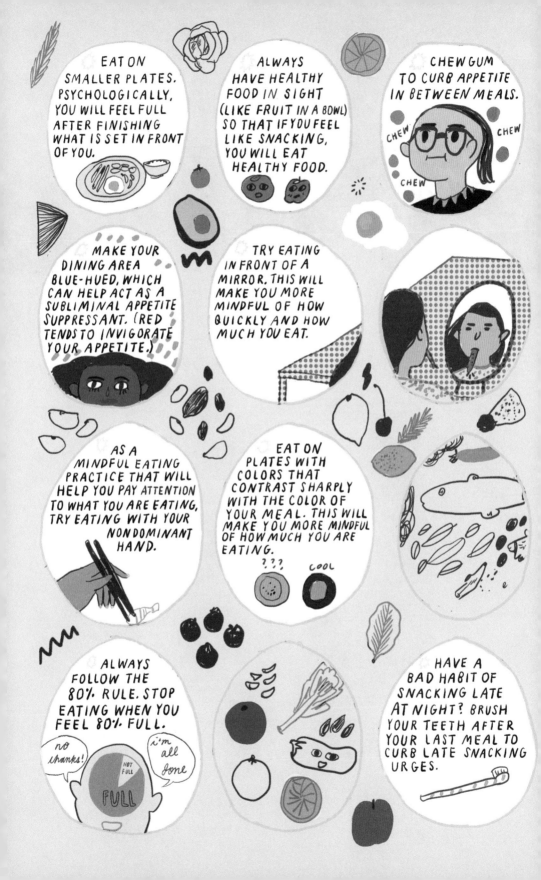

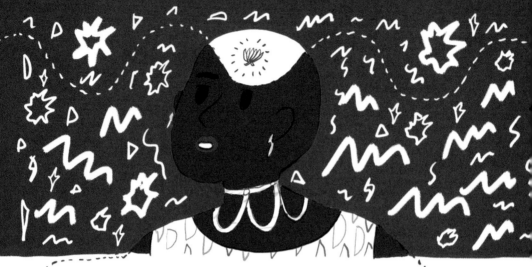

QUIRKY WAYS TO DE-STRESS AND FIND YOUR ZEN

⊛ DRINK ORANGE JUICE

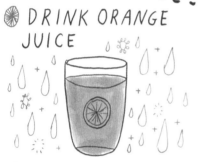

STUDIES HAVE SHOWN THAT VITAMIN C HELPS RELIEVE STRESS - AND BOOSTS YOUR IMMUNE SYSTEM, TOO.

⊛ GIVE YOURSELF AN EAR MASSAGE

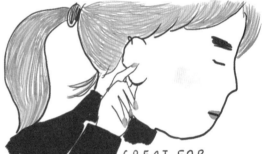

GREAT FOR HUMANS IN ADDITION TO CATS AND DOGS!

⊛ HAVE TOYS ON YOUR DESK

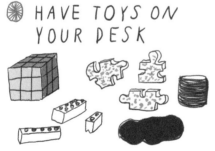

GIVE YOURSELF A MENTAL BREAK WITH KIDS' TOYS THAT YOU CAN PLAY WITH USING YOUR HANDS.

⊛ LISTEN TO WHITE NOISE

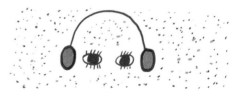

BLOCK OUT EXTERNAL STIMULI BY LISTENING TO WHITE NOISE, WHICH CAN HAVE A CALMING, GROUNDING EFFECT.

CARRY A WORRY STONE

FIND A ROCK WITH A SMOOTH SURFACE THAT FITS IN THE PALM OF YOUR HAND. ANYTIME YOU FEEL STRESSED, RUB THE ROCK WITH YOUR FINGERS AND IMAGINE TRANSFERRING YOUR STRESSFUL ENERGY TO YOUR STONE.

DO THINGS VERY SLOWLY

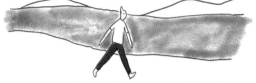

SLOWING DOWN THE PACE OF YOUR ACTIONS WHEN YOU HAVE A LOT OF THINGS TO DO CAN HAVE A CALMING EFFECT. EXAMPLE: DRINK TEA SLOWLY, TAKE A SLOW WALK, EAT YOUR MEAL MINDFULLY.

PRACTICE RADICAL GRATITUDE

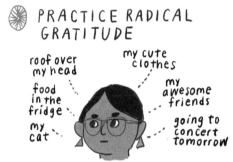

roof over my head
my cute clothes
food in the fridge
my awesome friends
my cat
going to concert tomorrow

MAKE A LIST OF EVERYTHING YOU ARE GRATEFUL FOR, FROM THE VERY GENERAL TO SPECIFIC, SILLY REASONS.

GO SOMEWHERE YOU'VE NEVER BEEN TO BEFORE

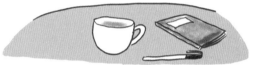

BEING IN THE SAME PLACE ALL THE TIME REINFORCES THE SAME THOUGHT PATTERNS, INCLUDING STRESS-CAUSING THOUGHTS. BREAK UP YOUR ROUTINE BY HANGING OUT IN A NEW SPACE.

DO A 10-MINUTE CLEANING BREAK

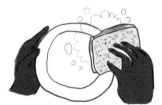

CLUTTER CAUSES STRESS. SET A TIMER FOR 10-15 MINUTES AND CLEAN YOUR SURROUNDINGS AS MUCH AS POSSIBLE. YOU WILL FEEL ACCOMPLISHED AND WILL HAVE MORE ENERGY.

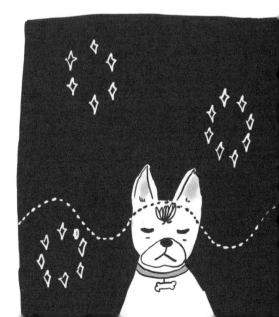

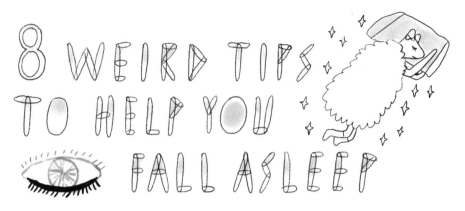

8 WEIRD TIPS TO HELP YOU FALL ASLEEP

◯ WHEN YOU ARE LYING IN BED, CURL AND UNCURL YOUR TOES.

◯ DRINK CHERRY JUICE. IT IS RICH IN MELATONIN, WHICH IN SOME STUDIES HAS HELPED ADULTS WITH INSOMNIA.

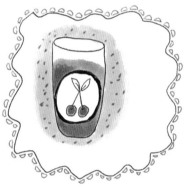

◯ 30 MINUTES BEFORE SLEEPING, HAVE A SLEEPY TIME RITUAL THAT YOU ONLY DO WHEN YOU ARE ABOUT TO FALL ASLEEP.

◯ RUB YOUR BELLY. STARTING AT THE NAVEL, RUB IN BIGGER AND BIGGER CIRCLES CLOCKWISE, AND THEN SMALLER AND SMALLER CIRCLES COUNTERCLOCKWISE. REPEAT.

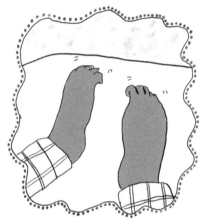

chamomile tea time

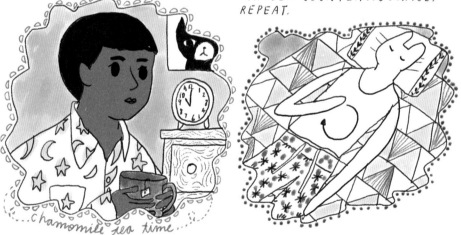

LISTEN TO WHITE NOISE, WHICH CAN BE AN EFFECTIVE WAY OF BLOCKING OUT OTHER NOISE.

THINK OF WHAT YOU DID IN THE MORNING AND WORK YOUR WAY CHRONOLOGICALLY THROUGH THE DAY. SOMETIMES THE MENTAL EFFORT OF REMEMBERING WILL MAKE YOU SLEEPY.

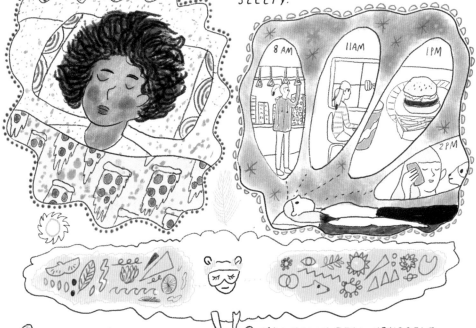

TAKE A COLD BATH OR SHOWER BEFORE GOING TO BED. LOWERING YOUR BODY TEMPERATURE WILL HELP YOU GET SLEEPY.

MENTALLY TELL YOURSELF THAT YOU ARE GOING TO STAY AWAKE FOR AS LONG AS POSSIBLE, WHICH WILL MAKE YOUR BRAIN REBEL INTO FEELING SLEEPY.

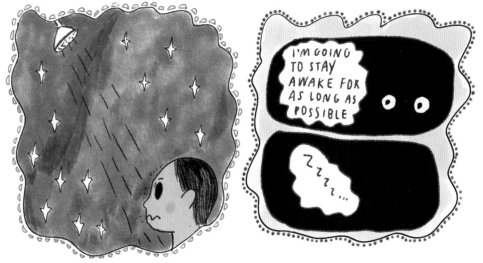

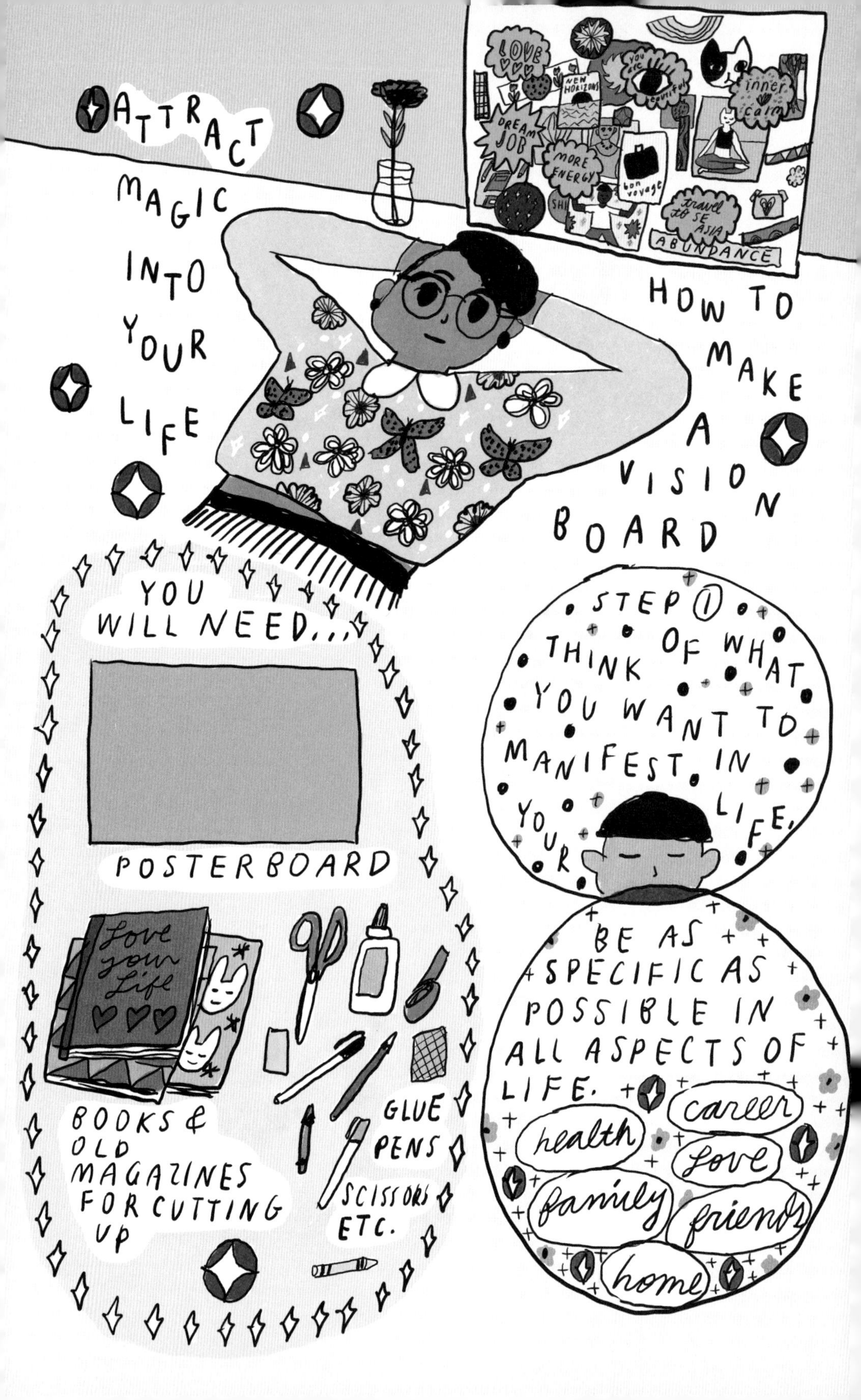

ATTRACT MAGIC INTO YOUR LIFE
HOW TO MAKE A VISION BOARD
LOVE
NEW HORIZONS
you are beautiful
inner calm
DREAM JOB
MORE ENERGY
bon voyage
travel to SE ASIA
ABUNDANCE
YOU WILL NEED...
POSTERBOARD
Love your Life
BOOKS & OLD MAGAZINES FOR CUTTING UP
GLUE
PENS
SCISSORS ETC.
STEP 1
THINK OF WHAT YOU WANT TO MANIFEST IN YOUR LIFE.
BE AS SPECIFIC AS POSSIBLE IN ALL ASPECTS OF LIFE.
career
health
love
family
friends
home

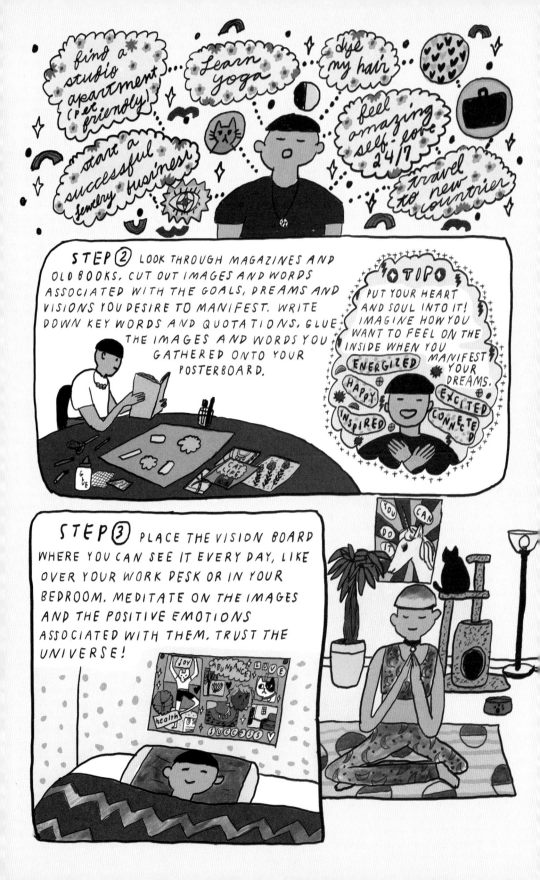

HOW TO FEEL MORE AWAKE IN THE MORNING

WITHOUT CAFFEINE

DRINK FRESHLY SQUEEZED JUICE (NOT FROM A CARTON). LIVE ENZYMES = MORE ENZYMES.

STIMULATE YOUR BRAIN. PLAY SUDOKU, DO A CROSSWORD PUZZLE, WRITE IN YOUR JOURNAL, LISTEN TO NEW MUSIC, ETC.....

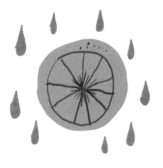
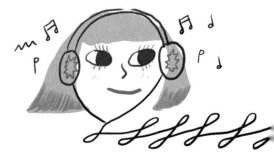

GIVE YOURSELF A DRY SKIN BRUSH BEFORE YOU HOP INTO THE SHOWER. USE A LONG-HANDLED NATURAL-BRISTLE BRUSH. BRUSH YOURSELF HEAD TO TOE. INCREASES CIRCULATION AND SKIN GLOW.

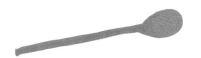

TAKE A COLD SHOWER, YOU WILL FEEL ALERT AND YOUR SKIN WILL FEEL GREAT.

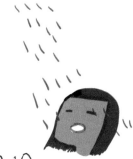

 EXPOSE YOURSELF TO DIRECT SUNLIGHT. THIS ALERTS YOUR BODY'S INTERNAL CLOCK TO WAKE UP.

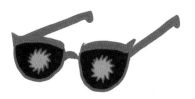

DO 10 JUMPING JACKS. A LITTLE PHYSICAL ACTIVITY CAN REALLY HELP!

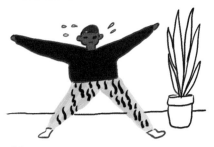

 TIDY UP YOUR SPACE. JUST 5 MINUTES OF DECLUTTERING WILL REFRESH YOUR MIND AND MAKE YOU FEEL ACCOMPLISHED.

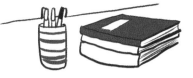

TIP
THE BEST WAY TO FEEL AWAKE IN THE MORNING IS TO HAVE A FULL NIGHT'S REST. DON'T SKIMP ON SLEEP!

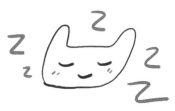

HOW TO TAKE THE PERFECT AFTERNOON POWER NAP

THE MOST IDEAL TIME TO DO A POWER NAP IS AFTER LUNCH BETWEEN 1-4 PM.

POWER-NAP IN A DARK, QUIET ENVIRONMENT. IF THAT IS NOT POSSIBLE, WEAR AN EYE MASK/ EARPLUGS.

KEEP YOUR NAP UNDER 25-30 MINUTES (IDEALLY 15-20 MINUTES).

19:59

DO NOT WORRY ABOUT FALLING ASLEEP. IF YOU CAN'T FALL ASLEEP, YOU CAN MEDITATE, DO BREATHING EXERCISES, OR LISTEN TO SLEEP-INDUCING AUDIO.

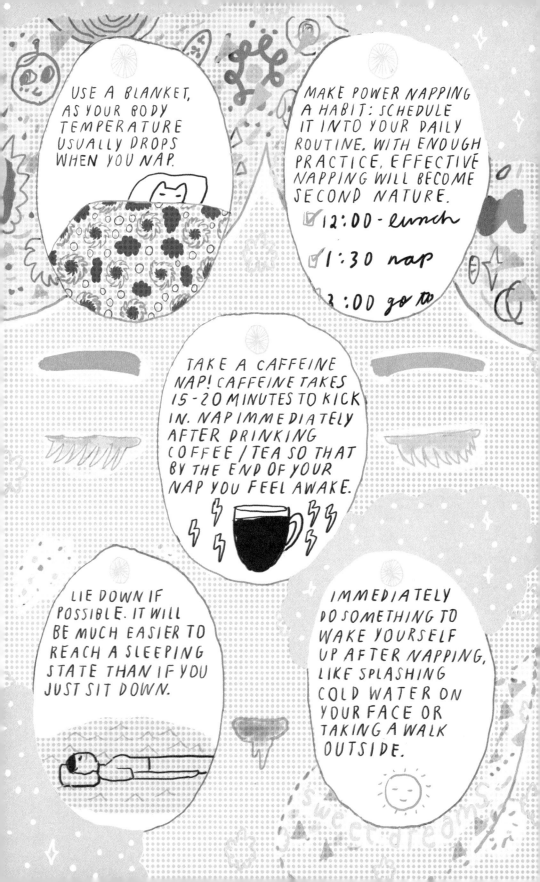

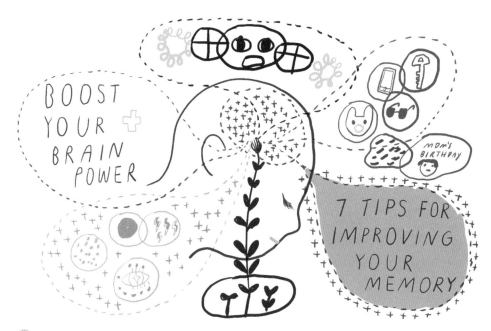

BOOST YOUR BRAIN POWER +

7 TIPS FOR IMPROVING YOUR MEMORY

⊕ YOUR LIFESTYLE PLAYS A HUGE ROLE IN THE STRENGTH OF YOUR MEMORY. DO THE FOLLOWING THINGS TO KEEP YOUR MEMORY SHARP.

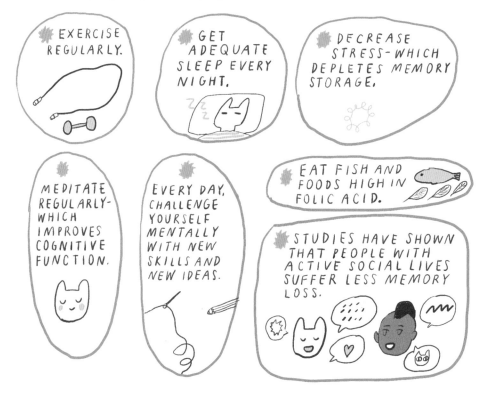

EXERCISE REGULARLY.

GET ADEQUATE SLEEP EVERY NIGHT.

DECREASE STRESS—WHICH DEPLETES MEMORY STORAGE.

MEDITATE REGULARLY—WHICH IMPROVES COGNITIVE FUNCTION.

EVERY DAY, CHALLENGE YOURSELF MENTALLY WITH NEW SKILLS AND NEW IDEAS.

EAT FISH AND FOODS HIGH IN FOLIC ACID.

STUDIES HAVE SHOWN THAT PEOPLE WITH ACTIVE SOCIAL LIVES SUFFER LESS MEMORY LOSS.

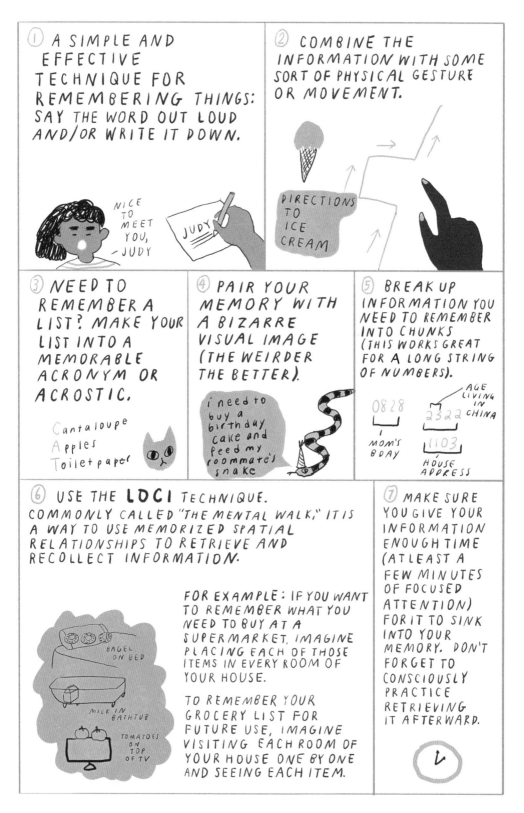

① A SIMPLE AND EFFECTIVE TECHNIQUE FOR REMEMBERING THINGS: SAY THE WORD OUT LOUD AND/OR WRITE IT DOWN.

NICE TO MEET YOU, – JUDY

JUDY

② COMBINE THE INFORMATION WITH SOME SORT OF PHYSICAL GESTURE OR MOVEMENT.

DIRECTIONS TO ICE CREAM

③ NEED TO REMEMBER A LIST? MAKE YOUR LIST INTO A MEMORABLE ACRONYM OR ACROSTIC.

Cantaloupe
Apples
Toilet paper

④ PAIR YOUR MEMORY WITH A BIZARRE VISUAL IMAGE (THE WEIRDER THE BETTER).

i need to buy a birthday cake and feed my roommate's snake

⑤ BREAK UP INFORMATION YOU NEED TO REMEMBER INTO CHUNKS (THIS WORKS GREAT FOR A LONG STRING OF NUMBERS).

0828
MOM'S BDAY

2322
AGE LIVING IN CHINA

1103
HOUSE ADDRESS

⑥ USE THE **LOCI** TECHNIQUE. COMMONLY CALLED "THE MENTAL WALK," IT IS A WAY TO USE MEMORIZED SPATIAL RELATIONSHIPS TO RETRIEVE AND RECOLLECT INFORMATION.

BAGEL ON BED

MILK IN BATHTUB

TOMATOES ON TOP OF TV

FOR EXAMPLE: IF YOU WANT TO REMEMBER WHAT YOU NEED TO BUY AT A SUPERMARKET, IMAGINE PLACING EACH OF THOSE ITEMS IN EVERY ROOM OF YOUR HOUSE.

TO REMEMBER YOUR GROCERY LIST FOR FUTURE USE, IMAGINE VISITING EACH ROOM OF YOUR HOUSE ONE BY ONE AND SEEING EACH ITEM.

⑦ MAKE SURE YOU GIVE YOUR INFORMATION ENOUGH TIME (AT LEAST A FEW MINUTES OF FOCUSED ATTENTION) FOR IT TO SINK INTO YOUR MEMORY. DON'T FORGET TO CONSCIOUSLY PRACTICE RETRIEVING IT AFTERWARD.

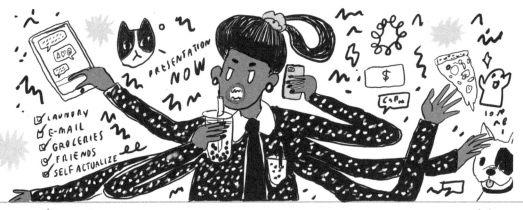

9 TIPS TO INCREASE YOUR FOCUS FOR GETTING THINGS DONE

USE A KITCHEN TIMER

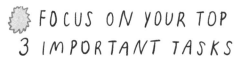

SET YOUR KITCHEN TIMER (OR PHONE) TO 30 MINUTES AND FOCUS COMPLETELY ON FINISHING ONE TASK UNTIL THE TIMER GOES OFF. (IF YOU ARE FEELING REALLY UNINSPIRED, SET THE TIMER FOR A SHORTER TIME - LIKE 5-10 MINUTES.)

BLOCK INTERNET DISTRACTIONS

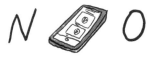

REMOVE DISTRACTING APPS FROM YOUR PHONE. INSTALL APPS IN YOUR INTERNET BROWSER THAT BLOCK CERTAIN SITES FOR SPECIFIC WINDOWS OF TIME. OR, JUST WORK SOMEWHERE WITH NO INTERNET.

FOCUS ON YOUR TOP 3 IMPORTANT TASKS

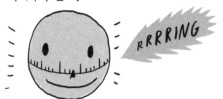

- ☑ WRITE 1000 WORDS
- ☑ FINISH PRESENTATION
- ☑ CLEAN OFFICE

PRIORITIZE YOUR TOP 3 TASKS FOR THE DAY SO THAT YOU HAVE A CLEAR IDEA OF WHAT YOU NEED TO FOCUS ON.

PRODUCTIVE PROCRASTINATION

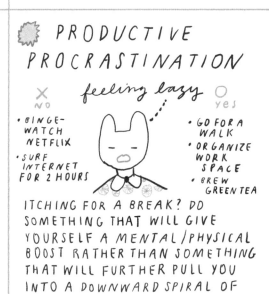

✗ NO   *feeling lazy*   ○ yes

- BINGE-WATCH NETFLIX
- SURF INTERNET FOR 2 HOURS

- GO FOR A WALK
- ORGANIZE WORK SPACE
- BREW GREEN TEA

ITCHING FOR A BREAK? DO SOMETHING THAT WILL GIVE YOURSELF A MENTAL/PHYSICAL BOOST RATHER THAN SOMETHING THAT WILL FURTHER PULL YOU INTO A DOWNWARD SPIRAL OF UNPRODUCTIVITY.

SET A SPECIFIC TIME TO CHECK & ANSWER E-MAILS

☑ 10:00AM

☑ 4:00PM

☑ 9:00PM

THIS IS FAR MORE EFFICIENT THAN ANSWERING AND READING E-MAILS ALL DAY LONG.

SET A CLEAR END TIME TO YOUR WORK SESSION

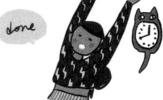

done

BY SETTING A CLEAR END TIME, IT WILL MAKE YOUR WORK MORE EFFICIENT AND FOCUSED.

SET A MINI-REWARD SYSTEM FOR TEDIOUS TASKS

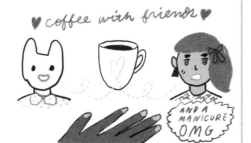

♥ coffee with friends ♥

AND A MANICURE OMG

THIS WAY, YOU WILL ASSOCIATE FINISHING A BIG TASK WITH SOMETHING ENJOYABLE AND FUN.

GET YOUR MOST IMPORTANT TASK FINISHED FIRST THING IN THE MORNING

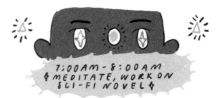

7:00AM - 8:00AM ♦ MEDITATE, WORK ON SCI-FI NOVEL ♦

GETTING YOUR MOST IMPORTANT (OR TEDIOUS) TASK OUT OF THE WAY WILL CREATE A POWERFUL MOMENTUM FOR THE REST OF YOUR DAY.

KNOW THYSELF

ARE YOU A MORNING PERSON OR A NIGHT PERSON? WHAT'S YOUR IDEAL WORK ENVIRONMENT? WHAT ARE YOUR WORST DISTRACTIONS? USE SELF-KNOWLEDGE AND SELF-AWARENESS AND EXPERIMENTATION TO OPTIMIZE YOUR IDEAL WORKFLOW.

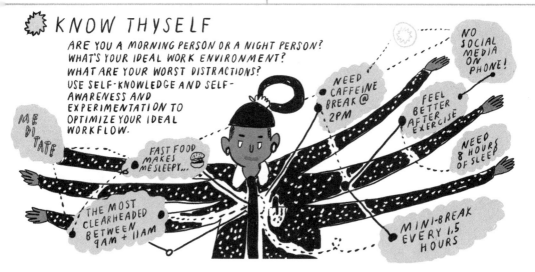

NO SOCIAL MEDIA ON PHONE!

NEED CAFFEINE BREAK @ 2PM

FEEL BETTER AFTER EXERCISE

NEED 8 HOURS OF SLEEP

MEDITATE

FAST FOOD MAKES ME SLEEPY...

THE MOST CLEARHEADED BETWEEN 9AM + 11AM

MINI-BREAK EVERY 1.5 HOURS

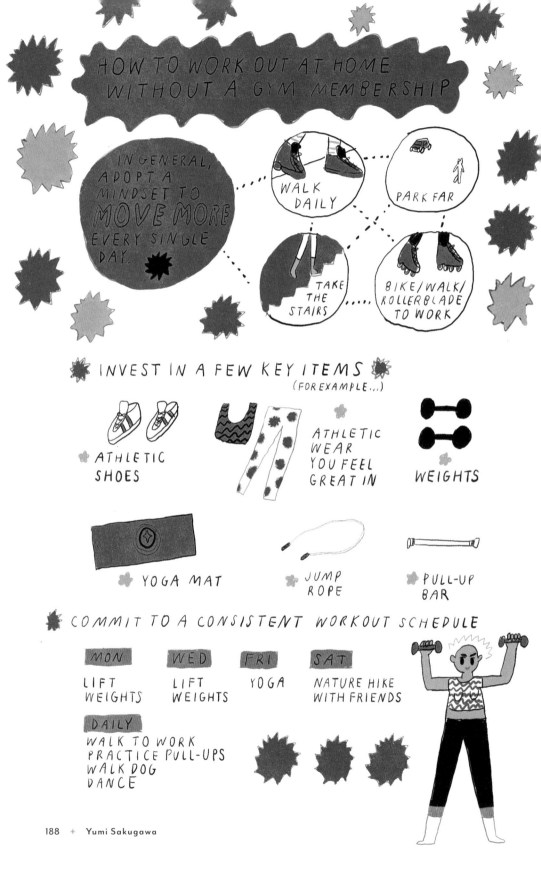

HOW TO WORK OUT AT HOME WITHOUT A GYM MEMBERSHIP

IN GENERAL, ADOPT A MINDSET TO **MOVE MORE** EVERY SINGLE DAY.

WALK DAILY

PARK FAR

TAKE THE STAIRS

BIKE/WALK/ROLLERBLADE TO WORK

INVEST IN A FEW KEY ITEMS
(FOR EXAMPLE...)

ATHLETIC SHOES

ATHLETIC WEAR YOU FEEL GREAT IN

WEIGHTS

YOGA MAT

JUMP ROPE

PULL-UP BAR

COMMIT TO A CONSISTENT WORKOUT SCHEDULE

MON
LIFT WEIGHTS

WED
LIFT WEIGHTS

FRI
YOGA

SAT
NATURE HIKE WITH FRIENDS

DAILY
WALK TO WORK
PRACTICE PULL-UPS
WALK DOG
DANCE

✸ TAKE ADVANTAGE OF THE FREE (OR SUPER-CHEAP) INFORMATION, RESOURCES, AND TOOLS YOU CAN FIND ONLINE / YOUR LIBRARY / APPS / COMMUNITY CENTERS.

PILATES VIDEOS

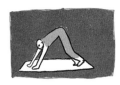
YOGA VIDEOS

EXERCISE APPS

EXERCISE BOOKS

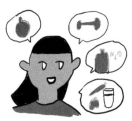
YOUR MORE FITNESS-CONSCIOUS FRIEND

LOCAL MEET-UPS

✸ A SMALL SAMPLING OF THINGS YOU CAN DO ON YOUR OWN WITHOUT GOING TO THE GYM

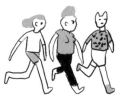

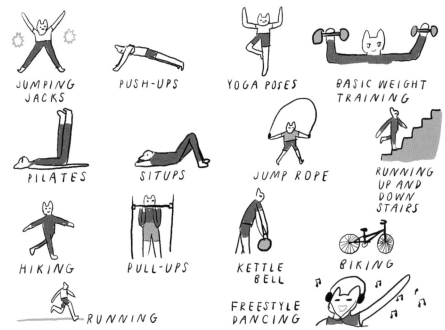

JUMPING JACKS

PUSH-UPS

YOGA POSES

BASIC WEIGHT TRAINING

PILATES

SITUPS

JUMP ROPE

RUNNING UP AND DOWN STAIRS

HIKING

PULL-UPS

KETTLE BELL

BIKING

RUNNING

FREESTYLE DANCING

MIND TRICKS TO ADD MORE EXERCISE INTO YOUR LIFE

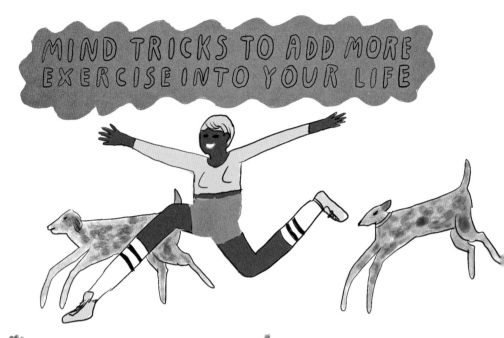

🌸 ASSOCIATE EXERCISE WITH A FUN ACTIVITY OR REWARD.

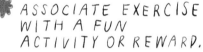

LIKE LISTENING TO YOUR FAVORITE PODCAST OR WATCHING YOUR FAVORITE TV SHOW.

🌸 BETTER YET, HAVE AN EXERCISE BUDDY AND MIX EXERCISE WITH FUN SOCIALIZING.

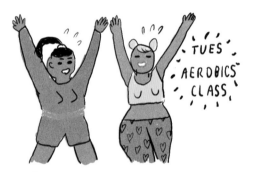

TUES AEROBICS CLASS

🌸 QUANTIFY YOUR EXERCISE/PHYSICAL ACTIVITY. LIKE...

90,000

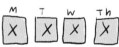
M T W Th
X X X X

MORE EXERCISE = MORE ENERGY

HAVING A PEDOMETER SO YOU KNOW HOW MANY STEPS YOU ARE TAKING DAILY.

OR MARKING YOUR CALENDAR EVERY TIME YOU REACH YOUR EXERCISE GOAL.

THIS WAY, YOU HAVE A TANGIBLE WAY OF MEASURING HOW EXERCISE BENEFITS YOUR LIFE.

SEE EXERCISE AS A MEANS TO EXPLORE NEW SKILLS, TRY UNUSUAL ACTIVITIES, VISIT NEW NEIGHBORHOODS, AND MAKE NEW FRIENDS. CHECK OUT ONLINE DEALS AND CENTERS THAT OFFER FREE CLASSES OR HEAVY DISCOUNTS FOR FIRST-TIME STUDENTS.

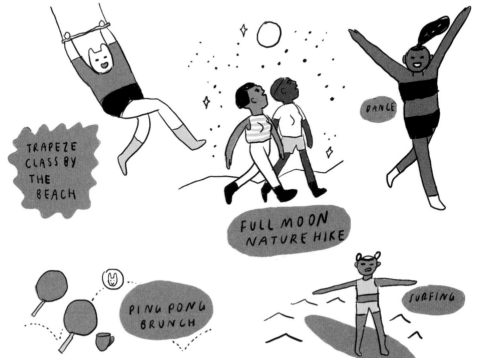

TRAPEZE CLASS BY THE BEACH

DANCE

FULL MOON NATURE HIKE

PING PONG BRUNCH

SURFING

SOMETIMES THE HARDEST STEP IS THE FIRST STEP. COMMIT TO PUTTING ON GYM CLOTHES AND WORKOUT SHOES. YOU'LL FEEL SILLY IF YOU DON'T FOLLOW THROUGH WITH EXERCISE.

HAVE YOUR OWN PERSONAL, POSITIVE, AND FUN REASONS FOR EXERCISING MORE.

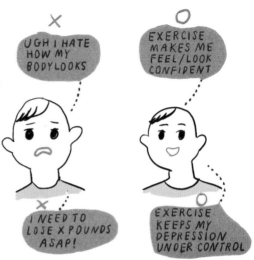

× UGH I HATE HOW MY BODY LOOKS

○ EXERCISE MAKES ME FEEL/LOOK CONFIDENT

× I NEED TO LOSE X POUNDS ASAP!

EXERCISE KEEPS MY DEPRESSION UNDER CONTROL

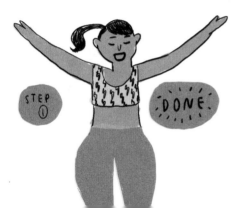

STEP ①

DONE

✻ IF YOU ARE HAVING TROUBLE COMING UP WITH MOTIVATION FOR REGULARLY EXERCISING, HERE ARE A COUPLE OF REASONS FOR YOU:

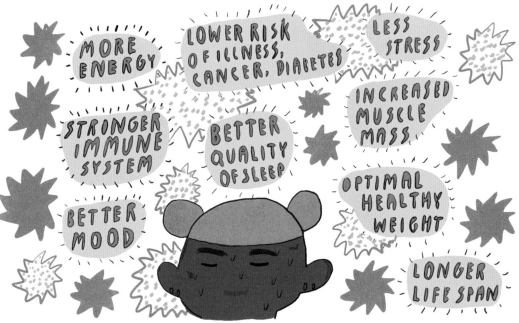

✻ PERIODICALLY REWARD YOURSELF FOR LEADING AN ACTIVE, HEALTHY LIFE. (IN THE END, BEING ACTIVE IS A REWARD IN ITSELF.)

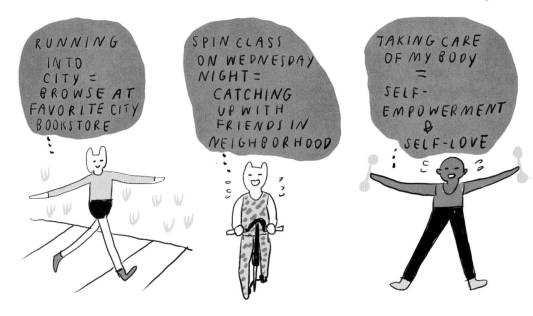